Reset Your
APPESTAT

Reset Your
APPESTAT*

A Successful Program for Achieving
Permanent Weight Control
Without Rigid Diets or Strenuous Exercise

*(ăp ə·stăt′) n. Appetite thermostat. The mechanism in the central nervous system that controls food intake.

by
BEN H. DOUGLAS, Ph.D.

QRP BOOKS
Brandon, Mississippi

Manufactured in the United States of America

First printing, April 1988
Second printing, August 1988

Library of Congress Catalog Card Number: 87-92249

Library of Congress Cataloging-in-Publication Data

Douglas, Ben H.
  Reset your appestat.

  Bibliography: p.
  1. Reducing—Psychological aspects.   2. Obesity.
I. Title.
RM222.2.D676   1988   613.2′4′019   87-29106
ISBN 0-937552-21-6

To

ALICE

for her exceptional support

and

JESSICA

for being wonderful

Contents

ACKNOWLEDGMENTS

The assistance of several people made this book possible. With their help, an idea was transformed into a finished product.

Birtice Boatwright searched out reference material and provided essential secretarial assistance. Pam Solomon, and other volunteers who used this method of weight control, identified parts of the program that needed clarification. There were several individuals who, after losing weight on the program, freely gave their permission to have their recorded conversations and weight loss data included in this book.

Working with the publisher was an enjoyable experience. Gwen McKee's tireless pursuit of perfection and Carol Mead's exceptional editorial ability were invaluable. Barney McKee kept track of a multitude of details, kept all else in perspective, and kept the project on course.

I am grateful to all of them.

About the Author

Dr. Ben Douglas is currently professor of anatomy, professor of obstetrics and gynecology (research), and director of the graduate program at the University of Mississippi Medical Center in Jackson. He received his doctorate in physiology and biophysics from that institution and was appointed to the medical faculty in 1964. He has been actively involved in teaching, research, and administration since that time.

He has published more than 250 journal articles, book chapters and abstracts of his presentations. His scientific articles have appeared in 28 different medical journals, including the *American Journal of Physiology,* the *American Journal of Obstetrics and Gynecology,* and *Endocrinology.* His particular research interest is the effect of the dietary intake of minerals and nutrients on blood pressure, body weight and atherosclerosis.

Dr. Douglas is a member of eleven professional societies, including the Society for Gynecologic Investigation, the American Physiological Society and the American Federation for Clinical Research. He has served as a review editor for several medical journals and is currently on the editorial board of *Clinical and Experimental Hypertension.*

Dr. Douglas has presented the results of his research before such diverse groups as the Polish Gynecological Society (Szczecin, Poland, 1980), the Society of Pathophysiology of Pregnancy (Dubrovnik, Yugoslavia, 1980), and the Japanese Hypertension Society (Sendai, Japan, 1985.) He has researched, written and delivered more than 100 scientific lectures to medical groups throughout the United States and to medical groups in Germany, Israel, Switzerland, Austria, the Netherlands, Ireland, Scotland, Italy, and Egypt.

Because of the significant data which Dr. Douglas' research has generated, he has received a number of honors and awards. Early in his career, he served for a year as a Visiting

Investigator at the Medical Research Council Blood Pressure Unit at the Western Infirmary in Glasgow, Scotland. In 1972 he was named an Established Investigator of the American Heart Association. In 1978 he received the American Heart Association-Mississippi Affiliate Silver Distinguished Achievement Award. In 1983 he received the Mississippi Academy of Sciences award for Outstanding Contribution to Science. He served that organization as president in 1985.

Dr. Douglas is the author of two medical books, and is a contributing author to four others. He is busy at work on a new book on how to slow down the aging process.

Many physicians consider obesity an incurable disease. In support of their hypothesis, they cite the multitude of unsuccessful treatments which have been used to eliminate this health-threatening malady.

Individuals who are overweight have been, and continue to be, inundated with diets, pills and devices which, their promoters promise, will bestow eternal trimness on those who use them. Few, if any, of the promised cures have proven successful. Aside from surgical intervention which forces a decrease in intake and/or absorption of food, virtually all of the methods which have been used to treat obesity have failed. Even surgery, with its associated risks, is not an acceptable solution to the problem of obesity for the millions in need of treatment.

Why do treatments for obesity so often fail? Do they fail because people who are overweight don't really try to lose weight, or because they don't care? Do they fail because people who are overweight have no self-discipline? Do they fail because people who are overweight have a flaw in their character? No. Those are highly unlikely reasons for treatment failure.

It's people who are overweight, not thin people, who carry around Tupperware containers of low-calorie food. It's people who are overweight, not thin people, who are constantly on diets. It's people who are overweight, not thin people, who are constantly going hungry. It's people who are overweight, not thin people, who are constantly searching for devices and potions to help them lose weight. In many instances it's the overweight person and not the thin person who is exerting the energy and making the conscious effort to be trim. It is an error in judgment to believe that an individual is overweight because of choice, lack of concern, lack of willpower, or lack of motivation to exert the necessary effort to lose weight.

Why *are* some people overweight while others are not? Simply stated, it's because that part of their brain which controls their food intake—it has been called the "appestat"—is set at a higher level than it is in people who are thin.

It follows then that a permanent "cure" for obesity entails either (1) a surgical procedure to *force* a decrease in food intake and absorption or (2) a resetting of the appestat. This book addresses the process of resetting the appestat.

It is not necessary to go hungry, go on a special diet, or engage in heavy physical activity in order to lose weight. People have lost weight without doing any of those things. Those who did used a more natural process to achieve the weight loss. They "reprogrammed" their body's appestat by doing some mental exercises. You can, too. The only thing that is required is that you *want* to lose weight!

This is not a diet book. There are plenty of those in print already. Hardly a month goes by without at least one diet book being high on the best-seller list. Most of the diets which they contain are simply variations of a basic, safe 1200-calorie diet. Some are not and are unhealthy. (Dieting or other weight loss programs in which you may be participating do not interfere with the process of resetting the appestat I will describe.)

The information which this volume contains is designed to help individuals reprogram their appestats. Once the reprogramming is complete, the appestat should automatically maintain the individual's weight permanently at the new level. People are hungry only if their appestat tells them that they are hungry. That is the reason it is possible to lose weight without feeling hungry. If the appestat is reprogrammed, it won't send out that message.

I want to share the Appestat Program of weight loss with you for a personal reason: Over the years I lost weight a number of times using various commercial and fad diets. I always regained the weight when I went off the diet (or when I could no longer tolerate the diet.) Finally, after the Appestat Program was developed, I used it to lose more than 45 pounds. I have not regained a single pound of that weight. I will never have to go hungry or count calories again. Neither will you when you use this method of weight control.

This book is to be *used*—not simply read and put aside. Mental exercises which are to be followed are described. Space is provided for scorekeeping. This permits a periodic evaluation of progress. You will be asked to keep a score, but you won't be asked to go on a diet at any time during this program.

Dieting is a fad whose time has passed. Diets not only don't work, they set individuals up to gain even more weight once the diet is discontinued. The reason for this is fully explained in Chapter 1.

Scientific information on related subjects, in readable language, is included. Various medical and surgical cures for obesity are outlined. Some of the commercial "cures" for obesity are discussed. The relationship of obesity to hypertension, heart disease and other problems receives special attention. Scientific information about studies on the effect of food intake on life expectancy and life span is included. Ways to prevent premature aging of the different systems of the body—and thus of the whole body—are described.

The way the body's different control systems work is discussed. An understanding of the working of the control systems of the body makes it easy to understand the mechanisms which govern body weight; makes it easy to understand why some people are overweight and others are not; and makes it easy to understand why reprogramming the appestat will result in permanent weight loss.

Conversations with individuals who are either still in the program or who have completed the program are included. These conversations provide insight into the way an individual's thinking changes as he loses weight.

The scientific information is included to reinforce one's *reasons* to be on the program. The scorekeeping, in addition to permitting an evaluation of progress, provides a part of the *repetition* necessary to establish new nerve pathways. The establishment of new nerve pathways is a necessary part of the process of reprogramming the appestat. The special significance of repetition in establishing these pathways is discussed in the introductory comments which follow.

This program of weight control is not for everyone. It is not for pregnant women, nursing mothers, people recovering from illnesses or perhaps others. *No one should undertake this or any other weight loss program without the advice of his or her physician.*

Ben H. Douglas, Ph.D.
Jackson, Mississippi

Reset Your
APPESTAT

Chapter 1

Introduction to the Method

Have you ever heard anyone say, "It isn't fair. He never goes hungry and he's skinny. I go hungry all the time and I'm overweight."? Every one of us has heard the expression. Most of us have used it. That's not surprising, since 62 percent of Americans are overweight.

Is it possible that 62 percent of Americans *want* to be overweight? No, they don't, and it really "isn't fair" that many weigh more than they should while there are others who maintain the proper weight without even thinking about it.

Suppose everyone had access to a dial they could turn to adjust their body weight to wherever they wanted it to be? They wouldn't have to diet, exercise, or count calories. Suppose they could adjust their weight just as easily as they adjust the temperature inside their homes. They could look at a dial, select the weight they want, dial it, then "set it and forget it." Then things would be "fair." Each person could weigh what he or she wants to weigh.

There are centers in the brain which tell individuals when to eat and when not to eat. (Because these centers control food intake, they have been referred to as the "appestat." That term will be used in this book when referring to the centers in the brain which control food intake.) Appestat, according to Webster's is "a neural center in the hypothalamus believed to regulate appetite." The hypothalamus is on the underside of the brain. It will be discussed in more detail later. By telling a person to eat or not to eat, the appestat controls the body weight. The appestats in different individuals are set at different levels. That is the reason for the wide variation in body

3

weight among people. The settings are different, but *they can be changed*.

If someone told you that you could follow a few simple steps to reset your appestat, what would your reaction be? Would you think that it could cost you several hundred dollars to learn how to do it? Would you think that you would have to go to a special training center and spend several thousand dollars to learn? The fact is, it doesn't cost anything to learn. You can learn the method and share the information with others if you wish.

Repetition is an important tool which can be used to reset the appestat. A word about repetition is appropriate here because it is an *essential* part of the process. Periodically individuals who are resetting their appestats will be asked to reread certain sections of this book. They will be asked to repeat a word or phrase a certain *number* of times—or repeat it continually for a given *period* of time. They will be asked to record a score daily after they say or do something which they perhaps said or did the previous day. There is a scientifically valid reason for doing this. Repetition is necessary to permanently establish, or change, nerve pathways associated with learning, memory, and other brain functions.

This phenomenon has been extensively studied. If an impulse travels from one nerve to another nerve in the brain, it obviously must cross a junction between the two nerves. If a lot of impulses cross the junction (repetition), the structure of the junction, the chemical enzymes within the junction and/or some other features of the junction change permanently. That makes it easier for other impulses to cross the junction. Once the junction changes permanently, a new nerve pathway and thought pattern are established. This provides a mechanism for the storage of information which we call learning.

When you learned your ABCs, you repeated them again and again. You didn't just take a cursory look at them and commit them to memory. The same is true for a multitude of other things that you learned. You used repetition to learn the days of the week, the months of the year and the multiplication tables. If you wanted to learn, or *permanently* store something for recall at a later date, you probably used the process of repetition to do it.

Repetition is a tool for acquiring new skills. The accomplished musician can sit at a piano and play a difficult piece, all the while chatting to someone. The fingers glide effortlessly up and down the keyboard as if the music was being played automatically. That type of learning and skill is acquired by endless repetition. New nerve pathways are permanently established by long hours of practice.

Temporary memory, which serves passing needs, does not require that the junctions between nerves be permanently changed, so it does not require as much repetition. A person can keep nerve circuits active for a short time—keep them "reverberating"—until a particular purpose is served. (Once a person has "remembered" to mail a letter, there is no need to retain the thought.) You want the resetting of your appestat to be permanent—not temporary—so repetition *will be required*.

Repetition can be used to achieve many things. Even new *reflexes* can be established by repetition. Humans are born with certain *natural* reflexes. The suckling reflex is present at birth. The startle reflex—sudden jumping in response to a loud noise—is present. Salivation in response to food odors is present, as are other natural reflexes. A new or *conditioned* reflex can be established by repeatedly associating a new stimulus with an existing one. Pavlov's classical experiments are an example. When he gave food to an animal, the animal salivated (natural reflex). He then rang a bell each time before he gave food to the animal. After this had been done a number of times (repetition), he rang the bell, but food was not offered. The animal salivated anyway. A new nerve pathway had been established. The animal had "learned" a new reflex; it had learned to salivate in response to the sound of a bell. With sufficient repetition, reflexes can be learned and the information stored in the brain.

It is likely easier to store memories in some parts of the nervous system than in others, but they can be stored in many different places within the nervous system. It is beyond the limits of the present discussion to include a detailed accounting of the evidence, but memory can be established in the "lower" brain centers such as the thalamus and brain stem. It can probably be established there about as easily as it can in the cerebral cortex or the "thinking" part of the brain.

Circumstances affect memory. Individuals tend to remember pleasant and unpleasant events. An attempt has been made to make the process of resetting the appestat a pleasant, rewarding experience. Repetition will be used in the process of resetting the appestat so that the nerve circuits will be permanently changed. Hopefully these nerve circuits will be as permanently established as the nerve circuits were when the ABCs were learned. It only requires repetition.

This program of weight control doesn't offer "something for nothing." (You should be skeptical of any weight control programs that do.) Some *patience* and *persistence* will be required in order for you to reprogram your appestat. The reward for reprogramming your appestat is that your body weight will *gradually* decrease until it reaches the level that you desire. Thereafter it will *remain* at that level.

Emphasis should be put on the word "gradual" because, as will be explained further, that is the way you want your weight to decrease. One participant in this program said that over the years he "grew up" and that by reprogramming his appestat, he was able to "grow down." Maybe his saying that he was able to "grow down" isn't correct word usage according to Webster's, but the message is clear. His body weight decreased gradually over a period of time just as it had increased gradually over a period of time.

We have all known individuals who, having slowly gained weight for years, want to lose the weight all at once when they do decide to lose it. Maybe they gained the weight at a rate of only a quarter of a pound a month but they want to take it off right away. (If they gained weight at the rate of a quarter of a pound a month for a period of 20 years, they gained a total of 60 pounds. It won't take them 20 years to get the weight off.

Using the Appestat Program they can lose two to four pounds a month.) However, human nature being what it is, that same person who took *20 years* to put the weight on often wants to get it off in *20 days*.

As a result he starts into a counterproductive cycle. He looks for a way to get the weight off quickly. He has visions of losing it in a few days, or at the most in a few weeks, then becoming his old slim, trim self again. He further fantasizes that after he loses the weight, he can go off his diet and live happily ever after; that he can eat whatever he wants to eat and remain trim as ever. It all sounds so logical. He decides to do it! He selects a diet which promises quick results. He loses weight—not the entire 60 pounds maybe, but he does lose weight. Then a vacation or a holiday season comes along. He "temporarily" goes off his diet. A few weeks later he steps on the scales and discovers, much to his dismay, that instead of being *60* pounds overweight, he is now *62* pounds overweight! What happened? He went on a diet and *gained* weight! After thinking about it, he reaches the conclusion that he simply used the wrong method of losing weight in the first place. He searches for a better diet—one that promises even quicker results. Little does he realize that the cycle is destined to repeat itself. Each time he will lose some weight, then gain that weight back plus a little more. His weight will continue to creep slowly upward. He might ultimately decide that going on a diet not only doesn't work for him, it makes him gain weight. Why does the cycle continue? There is a simple physiological explanation.

Severe caloric restriction causes a person to use up stored glycogen, a substance which is an important source of energy for the body. Much of the weight that is lost initially is not fat. It is glycogen and water. As glycogen is lost, the metabolic rate—the day-to-day use of calories—decreases. The body burns fewer and fewer calories each day, making it more and more difficult to lose weight. When the individual goes off a diet, it is easy to regain the weight that was lost because by then calories are being burned at a very slow rate. When a person goes off a diet, the glycogen and water that were lost are immediately replenished. The lost weight is regained. After replenishing the glycogen and water, the individual begins to store fat because the metabolic rate remains slowed for some time. The size of the fat cells increases. Not only does the individual's goal of permanent weight loss not get achieved, but the severe caloric restriction sets the body up for regaining the weight that was lost—*plus* some additional pounds—once normal eating was resumed.

When you reprogram your appestat, it will be done gradually over an extended period of time. Severe glycogen depletion will thereby be avoided. By avoiding glycogen depletion, you are less likely to slow your metabolic rate. As the appestat is reset, it will have you take in calories at a slightly slower rate than you use them (although you won't be aware of it). That will give your body time to adjust and "borrow" the extra calories that it needs from the fat cells in your body. The size of the fat cells will decrease. With time, the amount of stored fat in your body will decrease. Your weight will decrease while you maintain the proper level of glycogen and water in your body.

Since glycogen depletion and a decrease in the metabolic rate are avoided, resetting the appestat doesn't produce the malaise which an individual who is on a severely restricted diet might experience. To the contrary, individuals who work at reprogramming their appestat typically report that they feel "hyper" or "energized." They usually become more active instead of less active. The increased activity speeds up their metabolic rate both while they are active and for several hours afterward. Not only are they "borrowing" calories from their fat cells, they are using the "borrowed" calories more rapidly than they ordinarily would since their metabolic rate is up. The weight that is lost is not regained. They never "pay back" the calories which they "borrow" from the fat cells.

When you reprogram your appestat, you don't have to worry about what is going to happen to you when you "go off" a diet because you don't "go on" a diet to lose the weight in the first place. (And this is not to be critical of people who have tried diets. Many of us have. Millions of Americans are overweight. Over ten million are severely overweight. It is only natural that people who are overweight should search for a remedy to the problem. Much has been learned from those of us who have tried different methods of losing weight. New information is gained when people try things.)

People who are seriously contemplating resetting their appestats should be aware that they can do three things to accomplish the task. First, they can progressively acquire information about the mechanisms which control body weight. An accumulation of information allows one to appreciate the complex processes involved in permanently changing the body weight. It allows an appreciation of the benefits to be derived from making such a change. The second thing that they can do is use repetitious phrases. These help ingrain the intended message in the central nervous system. Third, keeping score enhances the repetitious process and promotes the implantation of the desired message in the brain. Keeping score may seem mundane and simplistic at times, but the act of doing it pays dividends.

Carry this book with you wherever you go. Follow the steps described in it. In addition to following the steps, *read **something** from this book before every meal*. When you do that, you are reminding your appestat that *you intend* to have your weight controlled at a new level.

It's only natural that you would have a lot of questions about controlling your body weight this way. Everyone does when they are first introduced to it. Listed below are some frequently asked questions about resetting the body weight control center in the brain.

Questions and answers about body weight adjustment.

Q. Does this method require a special diet?
A. No. The method does not require a special diet.
Q. Do I have to go hungry?
A. No.

Q. Does it involve counting calories or eating certain kinds of foods.

A. No. The method does not involve counting calories. It does not involve eating certain kinds of food. In fact, concentrating on food intake is not one of the features of this method of body weight adjustment.

Q. I have seen books which make the claim that they are not diet books. Yet, midway through them, recipes and a list of foods that one should and should not eat begin appearing. At that point I realize that they really are diet books after all. Is something similar going to happen with this program?

A. You don't have to worry about this book shifting gears after you get into it. This is not a diet book. It doesn't contain diets or recipes. It doesn't suggest that you change the type of food that you eat. It does *recommend* that you eat healthy foods.

Q. Doesn't diet have a role in the body weight adjustment method?

A. Only ten words need be remembered concerning diet: "Every person should eat a balanced diet every single day."

Q. Why don't you refer to it as "body weight *reduction* method?"

A. Utilizing this method, a person could adjust his or her body weight *up* or *down*. It could serve to increase or decrease the body weight. For that reason it is referred to as "body weight adjustment."

Q. What does a person need in the way of special equipment or foods to begin this program?

A. Nothing. It is not necessary to purchase shoes for running or walking, or clothing for aerobic activity. You don't have to purchase exercise equipment or spend money on special foods. It is not necessary to utilize yoga or special relaxation techniques, although you may be better able to use the necessary visualization if you are relaxed.

Q. How successful is the method?

A. All of the people who have completed this program have lost weight. That does not mean that as more people use the method, it will continue to be 100 percent successful, but indications are that it will be near that.

Q. How is it possible to lose weight without going on a diet or engaging in heavy exercise?

A. You change the setting of the appestat in your brain. The appestat then does the job it is supposed to do.

Q. Why are some people overweight and others are not?

A. This question relates directly to the one above. The "appetite center" in the brain sets a person's body weight by sending out signals telling a person when to eat and when not to eat. It does this to keep the body weight at a particular level. People who are overweight are not that way because they lack willpower or because they have a "flaw" in their character. They are overweight because their appestat is set at a higher level than it is in people who have a normal weight.

Q. Why do some people gain weight as they get older?

A. Their appestat remains set where it has always been and their metabolic rate—their day-to-day use of calories—decreases. (There is another, more complex, reason which will be described during WEEK SIX.)

Q. How is the appestat set in the first place?

A. It may be already set at birth. Identical twins who grow up apart from each other tend to have weights that are similar to each other rather than weights that are similar to those of other members of their foster families. This indicates that the appestat is the primary controller of weight although learned behavior—"clean your plate"—probably exerts some influence. The appestat is probably set very early in life.

Q. I have an important social event coming up in about a month and need to lose 25 to 30 pounds. Can I do that with this method of body weight adjustment?

A. This method of body weight adjustment is not a "quick fix" method. It is a method which allows your subconscious to gradually set your body weight to a new, *permanent* level—to the level you desire. Some time and patience will be required. To lose 25 to 30 pounds in a period of one month would require virtual abstinence from food.

Q. Wouldn't it be better to do that and go ahead and get the weight off in a hurry?

A. No. The weight would eventually be regained. The body weight would again go to that level set by the weight control center in the brain.

Q. There are a lot of special diets, programs and procedures for losing weight. How is this one different from them?

A. Virtually all diets, programs and procedures for losing weight have you utilize one of two common approaches: First, they have you try to *override* the weight control center in the brain. This means that you don't eat when you get hungry. Second, they have you attempt to *fool* the weight control center in the brain. That is, they have you consume large volumes of low-calorie foods such as lettuce, celery and diet liquids instead of calorie-containing foods. You temporarily "fool" your weight control center into thinking you have followed its instructions and taken in the proper number of calories. The weight control center will not be fooled for long. The current method is different in that you *reprogram* the body weight control center instead of trying to override it or fool it.

Q. Are there any commercial procedures which will result in permanent weight loss?

A. Yes, if you consider surgery "commercial." There is a surgical procedure which in lay terms is called "stomach clamping." The size of the stomach is surgically reduced so that the amount of food which an individual can absorb is reduced. This will result in permanent weight loss. Other surgical procedures are also used. They will be discussed later.

Q. Don't any of the other commercial methods work?

A. Yes, they work, but only temporarily. With rare exception they do not work permanently. There is a long history of individuals who have lost weight by one or a combination of those methods and then regained all of that weight at a later date. You can *override* the system for a short time but not permanently. You can *fool* the system for a short time but not permanently.

Q. If you can override it for a short time, why can't you override it for a long period of time?

A. Because the weight control center in the brain is more persistent than you are. It is set permanently, now and forever. It will maintain the body weight at a given level *until the setting* of the appetite center itself *is changed*. It works the way other control systems work. Here is an analogy from everyday life. Suppose the temperature in your house is 78 degrees. That is a little warm for you and you want to lower the temperature to 75 degrees. Instead of changing the thermostat on the wall, you decide to take another approach. You place a large tub of ice cubes in each room of your house. You position an electric fan so that it will blow air across each tub. The temperature in the house falls to 75 degrees just as you thought it would. It works; but remember, your thermostat is still set at 78 degrees. The heat will continue to come on. It will produce heat day after day if necessary. Sooner or later all of the ice cubes will melt. When that happens, the heating unit in your house will seize the opportunity to raise the temperature to 78 degrees, *exactly* where it was originally set.

You know of course that if you want to change the temperature in your house from 78 degrees to 75 degrees, you change the thermostat. The weight control center in your brain works the same way. If you want to change your body weight, you change the setting of your *appestat*.

Q. Can something similar happen with the weight control center in the brain?

A. Yes, it can. Here's how. You can *override* it if you don't eat. (Remember you haven't changed the setting.) You can *fool* it by substituting low-calorie foods and diet liquids. (Again, remember that this doesn't change the setting.) Then holiday festivities and other special occasions come along. You let down your guard a little. Your weight control center takes advantage of your being off guard and resets your body weight to exactly the level the weight control center has been programmed to set the body weight. You were able to override (or fool) the system for a while, but the system was more persistent than you were. The system finally set the body weight to where it was programmed to be set; to where the system thought it was *supposed* to be set.

Q. Is it possible to actually *change* the setting of the appestat?

A. Yes. A few simple steps and some patience are all that is required.

Q. How can it be reset?

A. That information will be given in step-by-step detail a little later on. In essence you will mentally use repetitious phrases to reprogram your appestat, acquire new information about weight control to help you understand the whole process, and keep score on what you do so you can evaluate your progress.

Q. Am I going to be thin after I read this book?

A. That depends on how fast you read it. If you read it in one afternoon and put it aside, you won't be "thin" the next morning. If you follow the very simple steps of reprogramming your appestat, your appestat will adjust your weight to a new level.

Q. When the stomach "shrinks", does that mean that the appestat has been reset?

A. After your appestat has been reset, your stomach might decrease in size in order to accommodate less food. If it does, you probably won't be aware of it. Resetting the appestat might "shrink" the stomach, but "shrinking" the stomach doesn't reset the appestat. (Surgically reducing the size of the stomach does not reset the appestat.)

Q. Where is the appestat or weight control center?

A. In a part of the brain known as the hypothalamus.

Q. Where exactly is the hypothalamus?

A. Picture this: Picture a balloon which is approximately half inflated resting on top of a hard-boiled egg. Visualize the half-inflated balloon as being the larger part of the brain, the thinking part of the brain, and the hard-boiled egg as being the thalamus. The hypothalamus is on the underside of the thalamus. The hypothalamus is a part of the brain that works somewhat "automatically." Now visualize a lot of connections between the hard-boiled egg and the balloon. This is a description of a crude model, but maybe it will help you to get the idea that the hypothalamus is on the underside of the brain. There are connections between it and the "thinking" part of the brain.

Q. Is body weight control the only function of the hypothalamus?

A. No. The hypothalamus has many important functions. It has a role in the control of respiration, blood pressure, and body temperature, just to name a few of its functions.

Q. No method of body weight adjustment is perfect. What is wrong with this one?

A. There is nothing "wrong" with this method. Some people might think that there are one or two things that need changing. First, the method seems too simple. Sometimes people are reluctant to try something if it seems too simple or too easy to do. Many people tend to believe that body weight adjustment must involve something that is complicated, something that causes discomfort, and/or something that requires a great deal of self-discipline. This method requires none of those things. A second feature which one might change is this: Because of the ease with which the appestat can be reset, some individuals might not remember to eat a balanced diet while it is being reset. If that occurs, the person should immediately correct the situation and eat a balanced diet or abandon the program.

There is one feature—the fact that the Appestat Program is inexpensive—which should not be changed, but it is a fact of life that if the method was so expensive that only a few people could afford it, some would find it very appealing.

Q. How can I lose weight if I don't go hungry?

A. You are hungry only if the appestat in your brain tells you that you are hungry. If your appestat is reset to a lower level, your body weight will be reset to a lower level automatically.. It will not be necessary for you to feel hungry in order to have your body weight adjusted to the level the appestat thinks it should be.

Q. How exactly does the weight control center in the brain work?

A. A detailed description of how it works is beyond the scope of this discussion, but basically it works as follows: In the middle of the hypothalamus is the center that lets you know when you are "full" or satisfied. It is the satiety center. If it is happy, you have no desire to eat. In the lateral part of the hypothalamus is the "hunger" center. When the satiety center

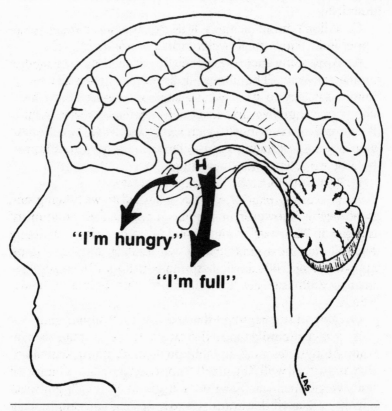

Figure 1. In order to control body weight, the hypothalamus (H) sends out two messages: "I'm hungry" or "I'm full." The visualization and repetitious phrases described in this book are designed to make the message, "I'm full," more dominant.

is not satisfied, the hunger center tells you to eat. This is a protective mechanism which insures the survival of the individual. If the satiety center is either destroyed or surgically removed, an animal will eat and never be satisfied. It will eat all the food it can for as long as it lives. It will literally eat itself to death. Thus the key to setting the body weight at a lower level is letting the satiety center know that it is "satisfied" at a lower level of food intake. It will be a subconscious adjustment. The individual involved won't be aware of the change in the setting. The change can be made relatively simply as will be described.

Q. I don't mind being a little overweight if there is an upper limit. How much weight can a person gain?

A. Apparently there is no limit to the amount of weight a human can gain. The human body seems to have almost an infinite capacity to store accumulated fat. Humans have been known to weigh five, six, or seven hundred pounds! Evidently it is possible to continue to gain weight until one dies. Weight gain beyond a certain point is referred to as "morbid obesity" because it becomes life-threatening.

Q. Can you "burn off" weight by exercise?

A. A sensible plan of exercise is an aid to well-being and good health. However, it requires a considerable amount of exercise to "burn off" one pound of body weight. Walking one mile for the average person will result in the burning of approximately 100 calories. An individual must burn approximately 3500 calories to "burn off" one pound of body weight.

Q. Does this mean then that exercise is not important?

A. No, it doesn't mean that at all. If the average person walks 15 minutes a day in addition to other normal activities, that individual will "burn off" approximately 12 pounds of body weight per year. That doesn't sound like much, but over a five-year period that translates to a total of 60 pounds. That doesn't mean that by walking for 15 minutes a day you will automatically be 60 pounds thinner at the end of five years. Remember the body weight control center in your brain determines your wieght. It must also be reset. If not, it might very well have you increase your intake of calories to offset those you burn while walking. But to answer the question, exercise *is* important. Do it, and be sure to do it sensibly.

Q. Okay, the method of resetting the appestat does not require a special diet, it does not require the purchase of special equipment, it does not require that a person go hungry, it does not require a great deal of self-discipline, it does not require that a person engage in heavy physical activity. There must be a catch. Is it going to cost a lot of money later? Is there some other "catch" to it?

A. There is no "catch" to it. It will cost nothing later. By simply repeating mental exercises, *you* can reset your appestat.

This is not a *fast* weight loss program as some other programs *claim* to be, but you must realize that this program is for *permanent* weight loss. It will take time and commitment. You don't have to diet, but you *do* have to follow all of the instructions in the book in order to change your appestat.

This program of weight loss might not seem fast, but a weight loss of two to four pounds a month will rapidly change your appearance. It is approximately the maximum rate at which weight should be taken off.

Q. Is it a challenge to reset the weight control center (appestat) in the brain to a different level?

A. Not really. It's easy to do. You can doubtless find enough challenges in your everyday life, so you won't be disappointed that resetting the weight control center in the brain is not a challenge.

Q. Should I reset my body weight two or three pounds below what I really want to weigh so I will have room to "vary" up and down some?

A. No. Don't try to "fool" your system. Set your body weight where you want it.

Q. Let's get to the bottom line. How fast can I lose weight?

A. You will lose two to four pounds a month until your weight reaches the new level.

Q. Isn't that awfully slow?

A. No. That is a loss of 24 to 48 pounds a year. In fact individuals losing more than four pounds a month should re-examine their food intake to be certain that they are eating a balanced diet.

Q. Can't a person lose weight faster than that on some of the commercially available diet/weight reduction programs?

A. Perhaps, but remember, as was pointed out above, there is a long history of people losing the weight and then regaining it. Let's consider two situations. See which one you prefer. SITUATION I: You get on a commercially available program. (The program may cost you *several hundred* dollars!) You lose 20 pounds in two months, then over the next 10 months you slowly but surely gain back the 20 pounds. (The weight control center doesn't forget. It is more persistent than you are.) Twelve months later, you're right back where you started. SITUATION II: You take steps to reset your weight control center, lose 24 to 48 pounds in 12 months and remain at that level. Which do you prefer?

Chapter 2

Getting Started
(Weeks 1–2)

Getting started is easy. Continuing through the different steps is just as easy. You can start at any time of the day, any day of the week. You follow a step-by-step, day-by-day, week-by-week program that will allow you to reset the body weight control center in your brain. You will know what to expect. You will have explanations for some of the feelings which you will experience.

Periodically you will be given scientific data and information which will reinforce your plans to set your body weight to a new level—to the level you want. This information is interesting and informative. It will give you better insight into the workings of the weight control center. It will let you know that the system is being reset. It will let you know that the system is working the way *you* want it to work.

Questions and answers will be included as you make progress in learning about the method. Scientific references will be included to document statements made; you may go to a medical library and read those sources if you wish.

You will need to keep this book handy so you can refer to it from time to time when you have questions. Read *something* from it before each meal. Take it with you to work! Take it with you on vacation! Keep it with you wherever you go! There are certain things you will wish to remember. You can refer back to them if you keep this book handy.

In getting started remember this: You aren't going to have to be thinking about *losing weight*. You *are* going to be concentrating on *resetting the appestat* in your brain. Then you are going to let the appestat do the job it is supposed to do. It is going to set your body weight to the level *you* want.

You can start the program at any time. For convenience we are going to assume that you are going to start early in the morning. That will make it easier to detail the sequence of steps.

During the first three weeks, the instructions will be given in step-by-step detail. You will find them a little more tedious to follow during the first three weeks than in subsequent weeks. By the time you begin WEEK FOUR you will be well into a routine. Some of the steps described may seem simplistic, but they are an *important part of the repetition process.*

WEEK ONE

Comments: *Carry this book with you today and every day. Read something from it before each meal.* Refer to it frequently so you can constantly bombard your subconscious with the new information.

You might want to put a part of the book on tape. Then if you find yourself spending a lot of time in your automobile, you can listen to the tapes while you drive.

Each week read the comments *for that week.* The comments are designed to provide a progressive buildup of information to match the particular phase through which you are working. Careful thought has been given to the feelings which you may be experiencing. For these reasons, even if you have read ahead, *reread* the comments for the week you are about to enter.

The steps which you are to follow during WEEK ONE are "conditioning" steps. They are covered in detail one by one because of the importance of conditioning you mentally for the resetting process. As time passes you will have an appreciation for the natural sequence of the steps. In the beginning you may feel the urge to "get on with it." That's okay; it may be an indication that you are ready to consume the new information.

Before beginning WEEK ONE, decide on a target weight. If your weight control center is going to set your weight to a new level, it needs to have a new target. It needs to know right from the beginning what that target is going to be. You, more than anyone else, probably know what your weight should be.

You probably shouldn't set your weight below your ideal body weight (IBW). The reference table of the Metropolitan Life Insurance Company is commonly used to determine IBW. IBW is determined according to sex, height and body build. You can approximate your frame size from Table 2 and determine your IBW from Table 1. Hopefully, you will always have this book with you so you can refer to the tables whenever you wish. However, if you happen not to have this book handy, and someone asks you about IBW, a rough rule of thumb for estimating normal body weight is as follows: For women, allow 100 pounds for the first five feet of height and 5 pounds for every inch above that. (If a woman is 5 feet, 6

Table 1
IDEAL WEIGHT*

MEN			
HEIGHT	SMALL FRAME	MEDIUM FRAME	LARGE FRAME
5'2"	128–134	131–141	138–150
5'3"	130–136	133–143	140–153
5'4"	132–138	135–145	142–156
5'5"	134–140	137–148	144–160
5'6"	136–142	139–151	146–164
5'7"	138–145	142–154	149–168
5'8"	140–148	145–157	152–172
5'9"	142–151	148–160	155–176
5'10"	144–154	151–163	158–180
5'11"	146–157	154–166	161–184
6'0"	149–160	157–170	164–188

Table 1. IDEAL WEIGHT *cont.*

MEN

HEIGHT	SMALL FRAME	MEDIUM FRAME	LARGE FRAME
6'1"	152–164	160–174	168–192
6'2"	155–168	164–178	172–197
6'3"	158–172	167–182	176–202
6'4"	162–176	171–187	181–207

WOMEN

HEIGHT	SMALL FRAME	MEDIUM FRAME	LARGE FRAME
4'10"	102–111	109–121	118–131
4'11"	103–113	111–123	120–134
5'0"	104–115	113–126	122–137
5'1"	106–118	115–129	125–140
5'2"	108–121	118–132	128–143
5'3"	111–124	121–135	131–147
5'4"	114–127	124–138	134–151
5'5"	117–130	127–141	137–155
5'6"	120–133	130–144	140–159
5'7"	123–136	133–147	143–163
5'8"	126–139	136–150	146–167
5'9"	129–142	139–153	149–170
5'10"	132–145	142–156	152–173
5'11"	135–148	145–159	155–176
6'0"	138–151	148–162	158–179

*Weights at ages 25–59 based on lowest mortality. Source of basic data: 1979 Build Study, Society of Actuaries and Association of Life Insurance Medical Directors of America, 1980.

inches tall her ideal weight would be 130 pounds.) For men, allow 106 pounds for the first five feet of height and 6 pounds for every inch above that. (If a man is 5 feet, 10 inches tall his normal weight would be 166 pounds.)

Since you now have a method for setting your body weight where you want it, you might be tempted to set it below your IBW. I don't recommend that you do that and I especially don't recommend that you set it more than 10 percent below your IBW.

Obviously age, body build, and other factors must be taken into consideration when you decide on what your new weight is to be. Take those factors into consideration and decide. *It is an important step in the resetting process to DECIDE what your weight is going to be.* DO IT!

Table 2
HEIGHT & WEIGHT TABLES

How to Approximate Frame Size

Extend patient's arm and bend forearm at 90° angle. With fingers straight, turn inside of wrist toward body. Place your thumb and index finger on the prominent bones on either side of elbow. Measure space between thumb and forefinger against ruler or tape measure. Compare with measurements listed on chart which indicate elbow widths for medium framed men and women. Measurements lower than those listed indicate small frame. Higher measurements indicate a large frame.

MEN Height in 1″ heels	ELBOW BREADTH	WOMEN Height in 1″ heels	ELBOW BREADTH
5′2″–5′3″	2½″–2⅞″	4′10″–4′11″	2¼″–2½″
5′4″–5′7″	2⅝″–2⅞″	5′0″–5′3″	2¼″–2½″
5′8″–5′11″	2¾″–3″	5′4″–5′7″	2⅜″–2⅝″
6′0″–6′3″	2¾″–3⅛″	5′8″–5′11″	2⅜″–2⅝″
6′4″	2⅞″–3¼″	6′0″	2½″–2¾″

Week One, Day One.

Summary of steps to be followed on Day 1.

Step 1. Weigh yourself and record the weight.

Step 2. Say to yourself *five* times, "I am slim and trim. I weigh _____ pounds." As you go through the book fill in the blanks with your *new* weight. If you are a male weighing 240 pounds and you are going to reduce your weight to 160 pounds, you would say, "I weigh *160* pounds." If you are a female weighing 170 pounds and you are going to reduce your weight to 115 pounds, you would say, "I weigh *115* pounds."

Step 3. At least 20 times during the day, at 20 different intervals, say to yourself, "I am slim and trim. I weigh _____ pounds."

Step 4. Each time during the day you see your reflection say, "I am slim and trim. I weigh _____ pounds."

Step 5. Read something from this book today.

Note. You will probably find it more convenient to repeat the phrases to yourself, but it is certainly okay to say them out loud if you wish.

Additional details regarding individual steps:

Step 1. Weigh yourself and record the weight. Weigh yourself early in the morning. You should not be wearing clothing when you weigh. Ideally you should weigh yourself three mornings in a row, and record the average of those three weights, since body weight can vary slightly from day to day, depending upon the amount of fluid in your body.

Q. Is it necessary for me to record my body weight so I can see that I am losing weight?

A. No. You *will* lose weight. You are recording your weight so if you start to lose weight *too fast* it will serve as a warning signal for you to reexamine your diet to be certain that it is balanced.

Step 2. It is important that you give your subconscious, or your appestat, the proper image. If it has the proper image, it will know where to control your body weight. Before you get out of bed in the morning, form a clear image of the way you will look when you have reached your new weight. Visualize yourself as the size you are to become. If your new weight is to be _____ pounds, visualize yourself as weighing _____ pounds. Visualize it as if you *now* weigh _____ pounds. Now say to yourself, "I am slim and trim." Repeat *five* times. It will take approximately six to eight seconds to do this. Now say to yourself, "I weigh _____ pounds". Repeat *five* times. This will require eight to ten seconds of time. *Constant repetition* is necessary to permanently change nerve circuits or establish new ones. If you wish, you may repeat this step at bedtime. That will give you additional repetition. You have just started your subconscious, or your appestat, on the way to forming the image that you wish it to have.

Q. Why don't I say, "I am *going* to weigh _____ pounds"?
A. You want to immediately start your appestat to accept the fact that you *now* weigh _____ pounds.
Q. Suppose I weigh 265 pounds and I want to reduce my body weight to 115 pounds. Would it be just as effective to say, "I want to lose 150 pounds"?
A. No. Again, you are *resetting* the weight control center in your brain (your appestat) *to a certain weight*. Now is the time to start to permanently place that image there.

Step 3. During the day, say to yourself, "I am slim and trim. I weigh _____ pounds." Repeat the phrase at random intervals until you have said it at least 20 times. Try to remember to repeat the phrase at least once each hour. If your business or occupation doesn't allow you to be that precise with your timing, that's okay. When you score your points at the end of the day, give yourself 20 points if you have repeated the phrase at least 20 times at 20 different intervals. If you repeated it less than 20 times, give yourself one point for each repetition.

Q. How will repeating the phrase help?

A. The sooner your subconscious, or your appestat *accepts* the image that you weigh _____ pounds, the sooner it will be reset at the new level. Once it is reset at the new level, it won't be satisfied until it has adjusted your body weight to that level.

Step 4. During the day, each time you pass a window, mirror or any other object which shows your reflection, say to yourself as you look at your reflection, "I am slim and trim. I weigh ____ pounds." This will reinforce the image formation in your subconscious. It isn't necessary to be absolutely rigid about the word "reflection." If you look into a mirror to see if you have something in your eye, or to see if your hair is in place, it isn't necessary to repeat the phrase. Repeat it when you see your *profile.* Also, if you notice something about the way your body looks—a bulge here or there—that you know is going to change, say to yourself, "I am slim and trim. I weigh _____ pounds."

If you do this on a *regular basis*—it may not be possible to do it every single time you notice your reflection or your body—give yourself 20 points at the end of the day. Even with your spouse around and your kids underfoot, you can silently and quickly say to yourself, "I am slim and trim. I weigh _____ pounds." (They don't have to know that you are doing something good for yourself.)

As your appestat starts to see you as slim and trim and weighing _____ pounds, it is going to start moving your body weight in that direction.

Step 5. Read something from this book today.

You have come to the end of the first day. You notice no mention has been made of dieting, calorie counting or going hungry. More importantly, you have started your appestat on the way to accepting the fact that your body weight is going to be _____ pounds.

Here is a quantitative method for evaluating your perform-ance. *This must be done every day, without fail, for the next three weeks for this program to work.* Give yourself 20 points for each of the following:

_____1. I weighed myself and *recorded* the weight.

_____2. I said to myself *five times,* "I am slim and trim. I weigh _____ pounds." I did this before I got out of bed. I did this while *clearly visualizing* myself at my new weight.

_____3. I said to myself at least 20 times, at different inter-vals, "I am slim and trim. I weigh _____ pounds."

_____4. Each time I saw my reflection during the day I said to myself, "I am slim and trim. I weigh _____ pounds."

_____5. I read something from this book today.

_____Total (Add 10 points to the total if you recorded your points on the day you followed the steps. Subtract 10 points if you recorded them at a later date.)

It is important to record your points. The *act* of recording points *provides repetition* and keeps you *thinking* about re-programming your appestat. If you accumulated 100 points, you are off to an excellent start. If you accumulated 75 points, proceed to DAY 2. If you accumulated *less than* 75 points, repeat the four steps in DAY 1. A point system will be given for each day that you are on the program. This is to allow you to judge your progress. You will need to average 75 points per day in order for the program to be effective.

Week One, Day Two.

Read something from this book today. Read something from it before each meal if possible.

A summary of the steps to be followed during DAY 2 of the first week of the program is as follows:

Step 1. Before you get out of bed in the morning, *clearly visualize* yourself at your new weight. While doing so, say to yourself *five* times, "I am slim and trim." Then say to yourself *five* times, "I weigh _____ pounds."

Step 2. At least 20 times during the day, at 20 different intervals, say to yourself, "I am slim and trim. I weigh _____ pounds."

Step 3. Each time during the day you see your profile in a mirror, plate glass window or other location, or you notice something about your body that is going to change, say to yourself, "I am slim and trim. I weigh _____ pounds."

Step 4. *Each time* you sit down to eat, before you take the first bite, say to yourself, "I *now* weigh _____ pounds". You may repeat the phrase to yourself during the course of the meal if you wish.

Step 5. Read something from this book today.

You will notice that the steps to be followed during DAY 2 vary slightly from those of DAY 1. It is important that you follow these steps rather than repeating the five steps of DAY 1.

Q. When I sit down to eat and say to myself, "I now weigh _____ pounds," is that to make me eat less?

A. No it is not to make you eat less. When you repeat to yourself the phrase, "I now weigh _____ pounds," you are sending a message to your weight control center. Remember, *you* don't have to be concerned about restricting food intake or about going hungry. You are only giving your weight control center a new image so it can do *its* duty. If *it* wants you to eat less, it will let you do so without having you feel hungry. If *it* wants you to eat less, it will have you do so and you will not even be aware of doing it.

As you follow each of these steps during DAY 2, keep in mind that you are reprogramming your appestat. To help you do this, *refer to the questions and answers of* DAY 1 (p.25).

Refer back to them at least one time. There were four questions and answers given. *Reread them.* Reread them more than once if you choose to and if you have the time. Remember, *repetition is important.*

You have now come to the end of the second day. Again you notice that no mention was made of dieting, calorie-counting, or going hungry. You may not be aware of it at this point, but your appestat is on the way to accepting the fact that if it does its job, it will be controlling your weight at _____ pounds. Your appestat is being reset.

Q. Suppose I suddenly feel that I really don't want to eat all of the food that is on my plate? I have always been urged to do that. Won't I have a tendency to continue to eat all of the food that is placed in front of me?

A. At the very beginning of the program you might, but later on you won't. Remind yourself that there is nothing more wasteful than eating something that you don't want or don't need. (You knew this already, but remind yourself of it—daily, if necessary.)

If you remind yourself of that fact daily and if you continue to have trouble leaving food on your plate when you really don't want it, try this: After you have finished eating, *purposely* put a small amount of some type of food on your plate and *leave* it just to see how you feel about it. Do this on several successive days. You will find that absolutely no damage will be done. Perhaps you were told as a child to "eat everything on your plate . . . think of the starving children in China." Maybe that thought is still in your subconscious mind, but you will find that not one single individual in the world will experience additional pain and suffering because you didn't eat something that you didn't want to eat. (Remind yourself that doing something that has an adverse effect on your health *couldn't* be helping someone else.)

Now quantitatively evaluate your performance on DAY TWO. Give yourself 20 points for each of the following:

_____1. I said to myself five times, "I am slim and trim. I weigh _____ pounds."

_____2. I said to myself at least 20 times, at 20 different intervals, "I am slim and trim. I weigh _____ pounds."

_____3. Each time during the day I saw my profile or something about my body that I wanted to change, I said to myself, "I am slim and trim. I weigh _____ pounds."

_____4. Each time I sat down to eat, I said to myself one or more times, "I _now_ weigh _____ pounds."

_____5. I read something from this book today.

_____TOTAL (Add 10 points to the total if you recorded your points on the day you followed the steps. Subtract 10 points if you recorded them at a later date.)

If you accumulated 100 points during the second day, you have the reprogramming process well on its way. If you accumulated _less than_ 75 points, _repeat_ the four steps in DAY 2 before proceeding.

Week One, Day Three.

Step 1. The first thing in the morning, _clearly visualize_ yourself at your new weight. Before you get out of bed, say to yourself _five_ times, "I am slim and trim." Then say to yourself _five_ times, "I weigh _____ pounds."

Step 2. At least 20 times during the day, at 20 different intervals, say to yourself, "I am slim and trim. I weigh _____ pounds."

Step 3. Each time during the day you see your profile or you notice something about your body that you want to change, say to yourself, "I am slim and trim. I weigh _____ pounds."

Step 4. Each time during the day you start to eat, say to yourself, "I now weigh _____ pounds." _Reread_ the question and answer relating to this step which was given on DAY 2 (p.29).

Step 5. Read something from this book today.

You are reprogramming your weight control center to set your body weight at a new level. You are going to have a new body weight. Write that weight down on a piece of paper and place it near your calendar, on your desk and/or write it on a piece of paper and use it as a bookmark in this book. In other words, place the number (_____) somewhere where you will see it frequently during the day. Each time you glance at it your subconscious or weight control center will be reminded that it needs to be doing the job that it is supposed to do and set your body weight at _____ pounds. It *will* do the job that it is supposed to do.

Give yourself 20 points for each of the following:

_____1. I said to myself five times, "I am slim and trim. I weigh _____ pounds." I did this while *clearly visualizing* myself at my new weight. I did this before I got out of bed.

_____2. I said to myself at least 20 times, at 20 different intervals, "I am slim and trim. I weigh _____ pounds."

_____3. Each time during the day I saw my profile or something about my body that I want to change, I said to myself, "I am slim and trim. I weigh _____ pounds."

_____4. Each time I sat down to eat I said to myself one or more times, "I weigh _____ pounds."

_____5. I read something from this book today.

_____TOTAL (Add 10 points to the total if you recorded your points on the day you followed the steps. Subtract 10 points if you recorded them at a later date.)

Week One, Day Four.

Repeat the five steps given for DAY 3 exactly as you did them on DAY 3. Sometime during DAY 4, read the following to yourself. If you have occasion to do so, you may wish to read it to yourself more than one time. (Repetition!)

"I am reprogramming my weight control center to set my weight at _____ pounds. The reason I keep saying that I am slim and trim and that I weigh _____ pounds is that my

weight control center needs a target. I am giving it a target of
_____ pounds. When I sit down to eat I tell myself that I
weigh _____ pounds to remind my weight control center of
the new target. If someone sees me eating less today, it is of no
concern to me. I am not dieting. I am not counting calories. I
am not going hungry. It does not surprise me that my weight
control center is doing the job that it is supposed to do. It does
not surprise me that I walk, talk, act and think differently. My
body is changing. I am supposed to feel the change."

Give yourself 20 points for each of the following:

_____1. I said to myself *five times,* "I am slim and trim. I
weigh _____ pounds." I did this while *clearly visualizing*
myself at my new weight. I did this before I got out of
bed.

_____2. I said to myself at least 20 times, at 20 different
intervals, "I am slim and trim. I weigh _____ pounds."

_____3. Each time during the day I saw my profile or
something about my body that I want to change, I said to
myself, "I am slim and trim. I weigh _____ pounds."

_____4. Each time I sat down to eat I said to myself one or
more times, "I weigh _____ pounds."

_____5. I read something from this book today.

_____TOTAL (Add 10 points to the total if you recorded
your points on the day you followed the steps. Subtract
10 points if you recorded them at a later date.)

Week One, Day Five.

Repeat the five steps given for DAY 4 exactly as you did
them on DAY 4. Sometime during DAY 5 read the following to
yourself:

"I am reprogramming my weight control center to set my
weight at _____ pounds. The reprogramming is underway. I
know my weight control center needs a target. For that reason
I keep reminding it that the target is _____ pounds. I have
the momentum going. I don't want my weight control center

to get lazy about resetting my body weight. The entire process is designed so that once my body weight control center is reset, my weight will automatically be controlled at the new level and I won't even have to think about it."

Give yourself 20 points for each of the following:

_____1. I said to myself *five times,* "I am slim and trim. I weigh _____ pounds." I did this while *clearly visualizing* myself at my new weight. I did this before I got out of bed.

_____2. I said to myself at least 20 times, at 20 different intervals, "I am slim and trim. I weigh _____ pounds."

_____3. Each time I saw a reflection of my profile during the day, or I saw something about my body that I want to change, I said to myself, "I am slim and trim. I weigh _____ pounds."

_____4. Each time I sat down to eat I said to myself one or more times, "I weigh _____ pounds."

_____5. I read something from this book today.

_____TOTAL (Add 10 points to the total if you recorded your points on the day you followed the steps. Subtract 10 points if you recorded them at a later date.)

Week One, Day Six.

Repeat the *four steps* given for DAY 5 exactly as you did them on DAY 5. During the first seven days of this program it is important that the steps be followed to condition your weight control center for new information which it will receive during WEEK TWO.

I want to encourage you to write your new weight down and put it in several places—mirror, desk, checkbook, calendar, and any other location that comes to mind. Then your appestat will be constantly reminded to control your weight at that new level.

This background conditioning is so important that if you have accumulated a total of 525 to 700 points at the end of the first seven days, you will be in an excellent position to proceed with the program. If you have accumulated *less than* 525 points at the end of the first seven days, repeat the programs given for DAY 5, DAY 6 and DAY 7 before proceeding.

This suggestion is strictly *optional*. If on DAY 6, while you are eating, you wish to say to yourself *repeatedly* "_____ pounds" (your new weight), then do so. (*Note:* If you choose to do this, don't let it influence what you select to eat nor the amount you eat. You are doing this for the *benefit of your weight control center* so it can then do the job that it is supposed to do.)

Give yourself 20 points for each of the following:

_____1. I said to myself five times, "I am slim and trim. I weigh _____ pounds." I did this while *clearly visualizing* myself at my new weight. I did this before I got out of bed.

_____2. I said to myself at least 20 times, at 20 different intervals, "I am slim and trim. I weigh _____ pounds."

_____3. Each time I saw a reflection of my profile during the day, or I saw something about my body that I want to change, I said to myself, "I am slim and trim. I weigh _____ pounds."

_____4. Each time I sat down to eat I said to myself one or more times, "I weigh _____ pounds."

_____5. I read something from this book today.

_____TOTAL (Add 10 points to the total if you recorded your points on the day you followed the steps. Subtract 10 points if you recorded them at a later date.)

Week One, Day Seven.

Repeat the five steps given for DAY 6 exactly as you did them on DAY 6. You may also elect to repeatedly say to yourself, "_____ pounds" (your new weight) while you are eating. This is optional and is not designed to change the type of food you select to eat or the amount of food you eat.

You have come to the end of the first week of the program. You notice that you have not been dieting. You have not been counting calories. You have not been going hungry. You probably notice that you feel a change. You should—your subconscious or weight control center is accepting the fact that a body weight of _____ pounds is the correct body weight for you.

Give yourself 20 points for each of the following:

_____1. I said to myself five times, "I am slim and trim. I weigh _____ pounds." I did this while *clearly visualizing* myself at my new weight. I did this before I got out of bed.

_____2. I said to myself at least 20 times, at 20 different intervals, "I am slim and trim. I weigh _____ pounds."

_____3. Each time I saw a reflection of my profile during the day, or I saw something about my body that I want to change, I said to myself, "I am slim and trim. I weigh _____ pounds."

_____4. Each time I sat down to eat I said to myself one or more times, "I weigh _____ pounds."

_____5. I read something from this book today.

_____TOTAL (Add 10 points to the total if you recorded your points on the day you followed the steps. Subtract 10 points if you recorded them at a later date.)

Add up your *total points for the week* and record:

_____TOTAL POINTS FOR WEEK ONE.

If you accumulated more than 525 points, the program is working. You are ready to proceed to WEEK TWO.

(*Note:* If you accumulated *less than 525* points during WEEK ONE, repeat DAY 5, DAY 6 and DAY 7 before proceeding to WEEK TWO.)

WEEK TWO

Comments: Before you start the program for WEEK TWO, please note the following: (1) New words of explanation or new information from the medical literature will be given to you during *each new week* of the program. (2) If there is to be a variation in the steps to be followed, the variations will be explained. The comments of this and subsequent weeks are designed to implant in your subconscious *reasons* for wanting to change your appestat. The repetition *changes* it.

As you begin WEEK TWO, remember not to go hungry in order to lose weight at a faster rate. Instead, concentrate on resetting your appestat. When you do think about food, try to think in terms of quality rather than quantity. Tell yourself that "bigger is not better" when it comes to food. Tell yourself that you prefer to concentrate on quality.

You can eat at home or dine out and still reset your appestat, but I would like to tell you about some feelings which have been experienced by others when they went into all-you-can-eat places. Their appestat reprogramming process continued to work but there was a mental conflict. They said that subconsciously they felt they were being urged, "get your money's worth." Even after they had eaten all they wanted, that small voice kept nagging at them to "get your money's worth." If you go to all-you-can-eat places, you might have a similar experience. (After you have been on this program for a few months, your appestat will be in control. You won't have to worry about the conflict.)

The following is a transcript of a conversation with an individual who has not been on the program long enough to lose all of the weight that she wants to lose. This particular subject has just completed the seventh week and is looking forward to additional weeks on the program.

Q. How long have you been on the body weight adjustment program?

Subject: This is the first day of the eighth week. I have completed seven weeks.

Q. Have you lost any weight?

Subject: Eleven and one-half pounds!

Q. That averages out to about one and one-half pounds per week?

Subject: Yes. That's about how fast it has been coming off.

Q. How does it feel?

Subject: Incredible! It's amazing because I don't even think about what I'm going to eat. I eat whatever I want and as much of it as I want. I don't ever feel hungry and I get on the scales and I don't believe it!

Q. So you are losing weight?

Subject: Yes. It's amazing. I still cannot believe it. When I get on the scales and my weight is down, I don't believe it because I'm eating all I want.

Q. But you know that is what your weight is supposed to be doing?

Subject: Right.

Q. How does it feel now that you have lost eleven and one-half pounds and you still have some more weight to lose? Do you feel confident that you'll continue to lose it?

Subject: Oh yes. I have no doubts about that at all. I don't even think about that anymore. At first I thought, well it'll probably work for everybody else but I doubt it's going to work for me. I've tried everything else. But I have no doubts at all now.

Q. Have you ever lost weight before?

Subject: Oh yeah, a bunch of times.

Q. What happened?

Subject: That (weight) plus a little more always came back.

Q. When you tried to lose weight again, was it more difficult than the time before?

Subject: Each time it was harder.

Q. So for a long time you gained and lost it. Your weight has been going up and down?

Subject: Right. Then I finally got to a point where I was putting on more weight than I was losing. I realized that I was losing ground so I said, "just forget it."

Q. Instead of losing ground you decided that it was better for your weight not to cycle up and down?

Subject: Right.

Q. Do you count calories or carry around calorie books?

Subject: No. I don't even think about whether the foods I'm eating are high in calories or not. In fact I've even eaten a banana split! And I've still lost eleven and one-half pounds!

Q. You haven't changed the type of food that you normally eat?

Subject: Oh no. I find that I prefer ice cream and chocolate— things like that—much less now but every now and then I still want it and I go ahead and eat it.

Q. So you haven't switched from the type of food that you've eaten all your life to things like carrots and lettuce?

Subject: No, not at all. In fact I haven't changed the menus that I prepare for my family. I still prepare the same thing. I just eat what I want.

Q. Do you think that this is the type of weight control program that other people could use?

Subject: Absolutely. Anybody could use this.

Q. Was it difficult to follow the different steps?

Subject: Not at all. In fact they are so simple that you don't really believe that they will work at first—because they are so simple to follow.

Q. So it doesn't require a lot of self-discipline?

Subject: It doesn't require *any* self-discipline. Not any! The only thing is that right at first it just required *remembering* to do it. Because you're so eager to lose the weight, that's not even difficult at all.

Q. Now that you're starting the eighth week of the program, do you feel that you have more energy?

Subject: Yes. I definitely do. I get up early (5:45 A.M.). In the past, at 8 P.M. I had to make myself stay up until 9 P.M. Now I'm staying up until 10 P.M. and don't feel tired.

Q. You feel more energized?

Subject: Much more.

Q. If you had to stay on the program for 8 to 10 to 12 months, do you think it would be a problem to stay on it for that long?

Subject: No problem at all. In fact if it had to be for the rest of my life, it wouldn't be a problem. . . . I will say one thing about the type of food that I eat. I find that I'm craving more fruits and vegetables than I used to. I think that I used to eat so much chocolate and ice cream and that sort of thing, that it nudged out my desire for the fruits. But now I desire the fruits over the other.

Q. Occasionally you have a craving for fruit?

Subject: Yes, for fruit. I've never had that before. I've never craved fruits before.

Q. What about your taste for chocolate and that sort of thing? I realize that you still eat it but has your taste for it changed?

Subject: Oh yes, I eat it now and then. I still have an urge for it but it doesn't give me the same satisfaction that it used to. It doesn't taste as good as it used to. It used to be that if I had a choice between fruit and chocolate, it would be chocolate every time, but not so anymore.

Q. Do you have any problem following the steps of the program when you go places—when you go to visit or when you go out to eat?

Subject: No, not at all except that I have noticed that in restaurants I tended to order too much food, but I've learned now not to have "big eyes." It's true. I would order what I was accustomed to ordering then I couldn't eat it.

Q. Are you going to reward yourself in some way when you reach the weight that you desire?

Subject: Yes. I'm going to spend *much* money on a whole new wardrobe and my husband is going to eat his heart out.

Q. Are you going to keep a big dress just as a reminder or are you going to throw everything away?

Subject: I'm going to keep one thing.

Q. Do you have any advice for anyone who might be thinking about trying this program?

Subject: All I can say is, "Try it." Try it because it works. It works one hundred percent.

The above subject is losing weight without following a regimented program of dieting and self-discipline. She will continue on the program for some time. That won't be a problem because, as she said, she could continue on it for the rest of her life if necessary.

Now, a word about scorekeeping. In order to conserve space, your score for WEEK TWO will be kept in an abbreviated form. The steps you follow will be very similar to those you followed during WEEK ONE. There will be a small (but *very important*) change in the fourth step. The first three steps will be exactly the same.

A word about **conflict** is in order here. As you practice the fourth step and say "I'm full," your hunger center and your satiety center will come into conflict. This will happen when you begin eating. As you say to yourself, "I'm full" during the first few bites, your hunger center may be urging you to "eat more." It may give you the urge to eat everything quickly. That's okay. Just say to yourself, "I'm full" as you chew, *pause after the first three bites,* have a swallow of whatever you're having to drink, say to yourself, "I really am full," then continue to eat normally. That will give your weight control center the opportunity to "balance things out" between your satiety center and your hunger center.

Here is a summary of the steps that you will follow *each day* during WEEK TWO:

Step 1. The first thing in the morning say to yourself *five* times, "I am slim and trim. I weigh _____pounds." Do this while you *clearly visualize* yourself at your new weight. Do this before you get out of bed. This step will be abbreviated "Get up, repeat (5x).

Step 2. *At least 20* times during the day, at 20 different intervals say to yourself, "I am slim and trim. I weigh _____ pounds." This will be abbreviated "Interval phrase (20x)."

Step 3. Each time during the day you see a reflection of your profile or something about your body that you want to change, say to yourself, "I am slim and trim. I weigh _____ pounds." This will be abbreviated "Reflection phrase."

Step 4. While you are eating, say to yourself, "I'm full." (More details about this step and the reasons for doing it are given below.) This step will be abbreviated "Meal phrase."

Step 5. Read something from this book each day. This will be abbreviated "Read."

During WEEK TWO give yourself 20 points for each of the following steps. Add up your daily totals. Add 10 points (bonus points) to the total for *each day* if you recorded the points on the day you followed the steps. Subtract 10 points if you recorded them at a later date.

KEEP YOUR SCORE FOR WEEK TWO HERE

Day 1	Day 2
__1. Get up, repeat (5x)	__1. Get up, repeat (5x)
__2. Interval phrase (20x)	__2. Interval phrase (20x)
__3. Reflection phrase	__3. Reflection phrase
__4. Meal phrase	__4. Meal phrase
__5. Read	__5. Read
__ Subtotal	__ Subtotal
__ Bonus	__ Bonus
__ TOTAL	__ TOTAL

Day 3	Day 4
__1. Get up, repeat (5x)	__1. Get up, repeat (5x)
__2. Interval phrase (20x)	__2. Interval phrase (20x)
__3. Reflection phrase	__3. Reflection phrase
__4. Meal phrase	__4. Meal phrase
__5. Read	__5. Read
__ Subtotal	__ Subtotal
__ Bonus	__ Bonus
__ TOTAL	__ TOTAL

Day 5

__1. Get up, repeat (5x)
__2. Interval phrase (20x)
__3. Reflection phrase
__4. Meal phrase
__5. Read
__ Subtotal
__ Bonus
__ TOTAL

Day 6

__1. Get up, repeat (5x)
__2. Interval phrase (20x)
__3. Reflection phrase
__4. Meal phrase
__5. Read
__ Subtotal
__ Bonus
__ TOTAL

Day 7

__1. Get up, repeat (5x)
__2. Interval phrase (20x)
__3. Reflection phrase
__4. Meal phrase
__5. Read
__ Subtotal
__ Bonus
__ TOTAL

TOTAL POINTS FOR WEEK TWO_____.

Week Two, Day One.

Follow the five steps that you will follow each day of WEEK Two and *record* your points in the space provided above.

Additional details regarding Step 4:
The first three steps and the fifth step that you will follow each day of WEEK TWO are now very familiar to you. *Step 4* requires additional comment: When you are on the way to breakfast, lunch or dinner, say to yourself repeatedly, "I'm full, I'm full. . . ." After you are seated at the table, say to yourself as you chew, "I'm full, I'm full. . . ." After you have eaten the *first three bites of food, pause completely* for a few seconds, take a swallow of whatever you're having to drink, say to yourself, "I'm full," then resume eating. **It is very important that you**

continue to do this from now until the end of the program!

During the course of the meal, say to yourself as often as you can, "I'm full, I'm full. . . ." You will find that you can mentally say the words very rapidly. You can say them as fast as you can chew. You will be able to say them to yourself and, at the same time, carry on a conversation with others who may be dining with you. When you have finished eating and get up from the table, pause and say to yourself, "I really am full." The rituals that you follow in Step 4 are perhaps the most important ones in the book. Get into such a habit of following them that they become a way of life to you. Follow them, no matter where you are or with whom you are dining.

Important: It is probably better if you don't eat between meals, but if you do have a snack, *do not* feel guilty. (Generally, "nibblers" are thinner than "gorgers.") As you have your snack, say the words "I'm full" just as you would during a regular meal.

Q. Do I say the words "I'm full" so I'll eat less?

A. No. You are simply reminding your appestat that it is perfectly all right for it to have you feel "full" at different levels of food intake. You should continue to eat normally as you say the words. (Remember you can't lose weight permanently by going hungry and overriding your appestat. You lose weight permanently by reprogramming your appestat.)

Q. Suppose I end up eating less because I say the words, "I'm full"?

A. It may be possible that you will end up eating less because you say the words, "I'm full" but if you do, *you won't be aware of it!* It will likely be impossible for you to know that you are eating less, although someone else might notice.

Week Two, Day Two.

Presume that you can learn something new. Resolve that you are going to work at acquiring new information and at resetting your appestat. You can learn new things because you do it every day. (The "thinking" part of your brain *and* the "subconscious" part of your brain can learn new things.)

Some adults claim that they can't learn as fast as they could when they were young. Is that because they can't, or because when they were young they automatically presumed that they *could* learn? When they were one year old they began learning a complicated language, they began learning the names of hundreds of objects, and they began learning new skills. Learning was probably made easier because the thought never entered their mind that they *couldn't* learn. Learning can continue throughout a lifetime.

During DAY 2, I would like for you to become aware of the exciting possibilities of learning new things. *Presume that you are going to learn something new!* Presume that your appestat is going to learn something new; that it is going to learn to operate from a new level. Get excited about the limitless information that is available to you! The following will help in that regard.

There was a time when a privileged few had a monopoly on learning. The reason was that books had to be copied by hand. Consequently, few books were available. Only the affluent could afford some of the ones which were available. During that dark period of illiteracy—a time when people didn't learn to read because there was nothing to read—one man had to work for 100 days to copy a book. Then in Mainz, Germany an inventive genius by the name of Johann zum Gamesefleisch, whom we know as Johann Gutenberg, developed a new method of producing books. He found that he could make individual letters out of soft lead and arrange them in such a way that they formed words, lines of words, and whole pages. That made it possible to print 100 books in a single day instead of a single book in 100 days. The world thirsted for and consumed the new information which was made available by the printing press.

Learning was no longer a monopoly of the privileged class. The printed word removed the last excuse for ignorance. For a small sum of money, people could acquire a friendship with the philosophers, historians, and novelists. (Today it doesn't even require a small sum of money. All that is required is a visit to the nearest public library.)

Gutenberg died in poverty, but we continue to take giant steps forward because of his invention. He discovered a way to make information available on a large scale. You have access to that information. You can learn whatever you want to learn.

The writings of scientists are available to you if you are interested. Medicine is no longer a mystical body of knowledge reserved for a privileged few. You can read about medicine just as you can read about philosophy and history. Even if you don't have a medical background, you can usually find medical information which is written in a readable language—as it is in this book.

Many of the ills which our ancestors regarded as inevitable consequences of living, or "acts of God," were diseases for which there are preventions, treatments and cures; or phenomena which have explanations. Once the stones of ignorance began to crumble, a flood of scientific thought surged forward. We have seen only the beginnings of the flood. Our lives have been permanently changed. They have been changed because learning is available to everyone. It is the monopoly of no one.

You can use that to your advantage. You can learn medical facts. You can learn to reset your appestat. *Know* in your own mind that you can learn to do it. Remind yourself of that frequently during the day today and every day. *Presume that you can learn.*

Follow the five steps and record your points.

Week Two, Day Three.

The use of visualization will be a part of this program of resetting your appestat. As you can probably appreciate, the various steps in this program of weight control were developed over a long period of time. They were revised, restructured, tried, and revised again until they evolved into their present form. When I followed the steps myself I was, after years of being overweight, finally able to lose the weight that I wanted to lose. I continue to use visualization as a part of the program. One of the things which helped me a great deal was the visualization which is described below. It is my favorite. I think it is a good attitude to have. It will help you too if you keep it in the back of your mind from now on.

The visualization is an attitude and way of life that an old civilization had. One night as I was reading about the habits and lifestyles of the ancient Greeks, it occurred to me that their attitude about eating was a good one.

The ancient Greeks believed in moderation in all things. Moderation was the ideal of their lives and not merely a hollow phrase. They were not enamored with having the "largest" or the "most." They believed more in quality than in size or amount. They built small but perfect temples. Their belief in moderation and quality could be seen in their clothing, their jewelry and their theater. They believed in a quality of living. They reduced life to a simplicity such that it became possible for them to enjoy leisure activities—the first time that leisure activities had been enjoyed by the masses in any civilization. The Greeks were neat and well-groomed. They believed in having a healthy mind *and* a healthy body. Their attitude about moderation and quality extended to their eating habits (van Loon, 1926).

When the family gathered to eat, the meal was simple. They looked upon eating as a necessity and did not allow it to take up a lot of their time. Eating was not a pastime with them as it is with us. They believed that spending too much time eating—and consequently eating too much—was a dreary act which produced dreary people.

When they ate they had some bread, a little wine, some green vegetables and occasionally a small portion of meat. When they dined with each other, which they loved to do, they came together more for the purpose of conversation than for the purpose of eating large quantities of food. Dining together was not the festive occasion we make of it. When they dined together, they didn't eat more than they should (or more than they wanted). They looked with disapproval on anyone who did. It is obvious that in this facet of their existence, they were oriented toward moderation and quality. (Even when a group of them gathered at a table somewhere to talk and to have some wine, they disapproved of anyone who overindulged.)

When you sit down to eat, think about the ancient Greeks. Think about their ideas of moderation and quality regarding eating. Think about them wearing their light togas and eating light food. Visualize youself as having the same attitudes. Say to yourself, "I eat because it is necessary. I like the idea of moderation. I like the idea of thinking about the *quality*, rather than the volume of the food that I am eating."

You are not using these visualizations and mental phrases to make you *consciously* eat less. (If you do eat less you will do it subconsciously.) You are using the visualization and mental phrases because it is a fact of life that *people become what they think about most!* Your subconscious will be motivated by your dominant thoughts. If you think about something long enough, that is what you will become. If you begin to walk, talk, act and think a certain way, you will reprogram your subconscious. Once your subconscious is reprogrammed, it will have you *automatically* walk, talk, act, and think that way.

Your subconscious will act according to the way it *perceives* reality! If it perceives you as a person who eats because it is necessary, who doesn't overindulge and who is interested in the quality of food eaten (instead of the volume), it will automatically have you behave that way. But first it must be reprogrammed. Once it is reprogrammed, it will take over. So think about those ancient Greeks and repeat the above phrases (often) about eating, moderation and food quality. Use the visualization and repeat the phrases to yourself, not just this week, but for as long as it takes to reprogram your subconscious.

Follow the five steps and *record* your points.

Week Two, Day Four.

Follow the five steps and *record* your points. Practice saying the words, "I'm full" *whenever you think about them during the day,* and especially whenever you feel the urge to have a snack. If you do have a snack, don't feel guilty about it. Just continue to work on resetting your appestat.

It is important that you feel good inside while you are resetting your appestat. If you have happy, exciting thoughts, that will make you feel good inside. That isn't exactly a new discovery, is it? The following idea isn't new either, but it was recently rediscovered (Dyer, 1977). Follow the logic carefully. There are three steps to it. (1) Since you feel good if you have happy thoughts, and (2) *since you control your thoughts,* it follows that (3) you can feel good whenever you want to feel good simply by having the thoughts you choose to have. *No one else* can control your thoughts *(unless you allow it)*.

Everyone around you can be moaning and groaning and flying in every conceivable direction, but *you can still think what you choose to think*. You can feel good inside if you choose to feel good. The rest of the world doesn't even have to know it. The world is going to keep right on turning whether your thoughts are happy or otherwise, so they might as well be happy ones. That puts you in control. Decide to feel good, then do it!

Succeeding at your goal of a new weight, a healthier body and a happier life is determined by *you.* Succeeding at it isn't a matter of being lucky or being in the right place at the right time. *You* are in the driver's seat. Get a firm grip on the wheel and make things happen the way you want them to happen. *Don't wait for someone to urge you to succeed!* You might have to wait a long time. Your life is a do-it-yourself project. It is *your* do-it-yourself project, so feel good and reset your appestat where you want it.

Week Two, Day Five.

Follow the five steps and *record* your points. Practice saying the words, "I'm full," whenever you think about them during the day.

It is important that you not try to starve yourself while you are resetting your appestat. You may be inclined to eat (or not to eat) certain foods in order to speed the process along. That isn't necessary. You should continue to eat normally and listen to your appestat as it changes. People might tell you that you should or shouldn't eat certain foods. You might read articles about foods that you should or shouldn't eat. When you get advice, whether from an individual or from an article, fact may not always be separated from fiction, so concentrate on resetting your appestat instead of worrying about what you should or should not eat. The following is an example of a substance that has been much talked about and much written about—and fact is not always separated from fiction in either the lectures or the writings:

A lot has been written about sugar and the adverse effects it has on the body. Let's take an objective look at sugar. About 11 percent of the calories in the average American diet comes from sugar. Sugar is a carbohydrate and, as such, is a source of energy. However, if you are eating a balanced diet, you are getting approximately 60 percent of your total calories from carbohydrates. That means it isn't *necessary* for you to eat sugar at all. Processed sugar, brown sugar, honey, and molasses are all different forms of sugar. They have calories but no vitamins, minerals, proteins, or anything else that is required by the body. It is true that if ice cream, candies, cakes, soft drinks and other sources of sugar were eliminated from the diet, a significant number of calories would be eliminated, but I hasten to add that it is not necessary to eliminate those things in order to reset your appestat. Once your appestat is reset, your appestat might eliminate some of them for you, but you won't care, and probably won't even notice.

Aside from adding unwanted calories to the diet, is sugar

actually *harmful?* No, it isn't. That is a popular misconception. It is not harmful in the quantities which are currently being consumed. If you have been eating sugar, you aren't going to have bad health because of it.

It is widely believed that sugar *is* harmful. That became apparent to me when I gave a guest lecture at a nearby college. Prior to the lecture a young woman (who incidentally was chain-smoking cigarettes) told me about the harmful effects of sugar—about how it causes everything from hardening of the arteries to diabetes to high blood pressure.

In a recent report, the Food and Drug Administration's Sugar Task Force disputes beliefs such as these. (You may buy the complete report for $15 from the American Institute of Nutrition, 9650 Rockville Pike, Bethesda, MD 20814.) The task force concluded that the amount of added sugar in the average diet does not contribute to any serious health problems other than dental cavities. (That doesn't automatically mean that it would be safe to eat large quantities of sugar.)

The report concluded that sugar in the amount currently being consumed does not cause diabetes, high blood pressure, blood lipid problems, heart and blood vessel disease, behavioral problems, obesity, gallstones, nutritional deficiences or a tendency to get cancer. (Note: The fact that sugar doesn't *cause* diabetes doesn't mean that, if you are a diabetic, you can begin eating all the sugar you want. In order to effectively control this disease, you should use the medication and follow the dietary guidelines prescribed by your physician.)

What *does* sugar do? It adds calories and quick energy but adds nothing that is essential for body function.

By the time you complete this program, you may be eating less sugar than you did in the past. Your appestat will likely change your eating habits without your knowing it. In the meantime, follow the steps outlined in this program. You want to concentrate on resetting your appestat so that your body weight can be controlled by your appestat.

Week Two, Day Six.

Follow the *five steps* and *record* your points. (Remember it is just as important to say, "I am slim and trim. I weigh _____ pounds" as it is to say "I'm full.") Keep in mind that you are becoming healthier as your weight decreases.

As your weight decreases you are helping your heart and blood vessels (more about that in Chapter 5.) People develop heart and blood vessel diseases faster if their blood cholesterol levels are high. By reducing your weight you are changing your blood cholesterol levels. Cholesterol has been much in the news in recent years. As a result of a new discovery, there is some good news about controlling cholesterol.

Cholesterol is present in the diet of almost everyone. It can be absorbed directly from the intestine without previous digestion. The body also produces cholesterol. Thus the cholesterol in the blood comes from two sources: that which is in the diet and that which the body manufactures. The basic nucleus of cholesterol is used by the body as a building block to make hormones.

Although cholesterol is useful, too much of it is not good for the body. The blood cholesterol level will rise if a person eats too much cholesterol, eats too many saturated fats, has thyroid problems (low amounts of thyroid hormone), or has diabetes. Normally the liver regulates the amount of cholesterol in the blood. It can manufacture cholesterol or take cholesterol out of the blood. The liver has "receptors" for cholesterol to take it out of the blood. But if the liver doesn't have enough receptors or if there is too much cholesterol in the blood for the liver to handle, the blood cholesterol levels will remain high.

People have become aware that a proper diet can reduce blood cholesterol. According to the *Journal of the American Medical Association* (February, 1987), men have reduced their blood cholesterol through dietary adjustments from 217 to 211 and women reduced theirs from 223 to 215. These values are within the normal range, and physicians don't ordinarily prescribe treatment for individuals whose blood cholesterol ranges from 200 to 220. Continued good dietary habits will probably cause the blood cholesterol levels of both men and women to decrease even further. That's good. In my opinion, the current levels are too high.

Proper eating habits can reduce the blood cholesterol levels in most individuals, but some people have a hereditary condition that causes them to have high blood cholesterol levels. This condition does not respond well to diets. Diets won't bring the blood cholesterol of these individuals back to a desired level. But there is a new cholesterol-lowering drug which apparently can.

The trade name of the drug is Mevacor. It is expected to be widely used. Mevacor could help prevent thousands of deaths from heart and blood vessel disease. (Consult your physician about this.) The discovery of Mevacor makes two options available to individuals: Those with only slightly elevated blood cholesterol can lower theirs by eating the proper foods, and those with unusually high blood cholesterol levels can take medication for the condition.

Week Two, Day Seven.

Follow the five steps and *record* your points. Reread the instructions given on DAY 2 of this week. Presume that any part of your brain—including your appestat—can acquire new information.

Congratulations, you have now come to the end of WEEK TWO. You are *well* on the way to resetting your appestat to a *new* and *permanent* level.

(If you accumulated *more than* 525 points during WEEK TWO, you are in an excellent position to continue. If you accumulated *less than* 500 points during WEEK TWO, *repeat* the steps for WEEK TWO before proceeding.)

Chapter 3

Understanding
and Eliminating Obesity
(Weeks 3–6)

WEEK THREE

Comments: You are about to begin WEEK THREE. If you haven't done so already, you will probably find yourself attending some special function and eating more food than you would have eaten had you not attended. (As a matter of fact this is highly likely since eating is something of a pastime with Americans.) If this does happen to you, don't feel guilty about "temporarily going off the program." *You didn't go off the program* if you continued to repeat the phrases and use the visualization. Rather than feel guilty, realize that resetting the appestat is a *gradual* process. It doesn't happen overnight. A year from now when you attend that same function, you will eat what your appestat tells you to eat and you won't even be aware that you are doing it. Just remember to be persistent in your efforts to change your appestat, rather than using some of your energy feeling guilty. If you have a tendency to feel guilty, turn right now to the comments of WEEK SEVENTEEN (page 108) and read about what feeling guilty can accomplish (or rather what it *doesn't* accomplish). After you do that, read what the individual below has to say.

The following was taken from a recording. The statements are verbatim and unedited:

54

I couldn't believe it. I stepped on the scales and they said 142. I thought for a second they must be wrong . . . I knew they weren't though. I had been saying 142 to myself for about ten months or so. Now the scales were saying the same thing. I'd been overweight for 30 years—not much . . . I thought not much. I'd been as much as 41 pounds heavier than I was in high school and college. People seemed to think that was normal. Most all men get a middle-age spread. It might have seemed normal but I didn't particularly like the way it looked. I missed the way I used to look. I'd look at my high school and college pictures and see I had a trim waist and would want it to be again. . . . One time or another I'd used about all the weight-losing plans. I'd lose a lot of weight but then put it all back on. Now I weigh 142 and it seems like I didn't have anything to do with it. I felt kinda guilty. Here I'd lost all this weight and I hadn't even been on a diet. I wanted to say, "look what I've done" but I really didn't feel like I'd done it. I still eat and I'm still full but now I weigh about what I did in high school and college. It's funny the scales said 142. They didn't say 141 or 143.

KEEP YOUR SCORE FOR WEEK THREE HERE

During WEEK THREE give yourself 20 points for each of the following steps. Add up your daily totals. Add 10 points (bonus points) to the total for *each day* if you recorded your points on the day you followed the steps. Subtract 10 points if you recorded them at a later date.

Day 1	Day 2
__1. Get up, repeat (5x)	__1. Get up, repeat (5x)
__2. Interval phrase (20x)	__2. Interval phrase (20x)
__3. Reflection phrase	__3. Reflection phrase
__4. Meal phrase	__4. Meal phrase
__5. Read	__5. Read
__ Subtotal	__ Subtotal
__ Bonus	__ Bonus
__ TOTAL	__ TOTAL

Day 3

__1. Get up, repeat (5x)
__2. Interval phrase (20x)
__3. Reflection phrase
__4. Meal phrase
__5. Read
__ Subtotal
__ Bonus
__ TOTAL

Day 4

__1. Get up, repeat (5x)
__2. Interval phrase (20x)
__3. Reflection phrase
__4. Meal phrase
__5. Read
__ Subtotal
__ Bonus
__ TOTAL

Day 5

__1. Get up, repeat (5x)
__2. Interval phrase (20x)
__3. Reflection phrase
__4. Meal phrase
__5. Read
__ Subtotal
__ Bonus
__ TOTAL

Day 6

__1. Get up, repeat (5x)
__2. Interval phrase (20x)
__3. Reflection phrase
__4. Meal phrase
__5. Read
__ Subtotal
__ Bonus
__ TOTAL

Day 7

__1. Get up, repeat (5x)
__2. Interval phrase (20x)
__3. Reflection phrase
__4. Meal phrase
__5. Read
__ Subtotal
__ Bonus
__ TOTAL

TOTAL POINTS FOR WEEK THREE_____.

Week Three, Day One.

Follow the five steps carefully. *Record* your points for the day. At the end of the day *reread* the unedited statements taken from the recording by the individual whose weight was reset at 142 pounds (p.55).

Week Three, Day Two.

Follow the five steps carefully. *Record* your points for the day. In addition to following the steps, tell yourself that you are intrigued by the idea of moderation in living, including dietary moderation. Practice this all day long.

Week Three, Day Three.

Follow the five steps carefully. *Record* your points for the day. Remind yourself that there is a *reason* (repetition!) for following each step correctly. Today, reread the special section about the ancient Greeks (p.47).

Week Three, Day Four.

Follow the five steps carefully. *Record* your points for the day. Be sure to say "I'm full" while you are eating. This is *most* important.

Q. Instead of saying, "I'm full," would it be just as effective to say, "I'm not hungry"?

A. No, definitely not. Your subconscious, or weight control center, might pick up on the word "hungry" and delay the resetting process. Say, "I'm full."

Week Three, Day Five.

Follow the five steps carefully. *Record* your points for the day. Today, remind yourself continually that moderation is rewarding.

Week Three, Day Six.

Follow the five steps carefully. *Record* your points for the day.

Week Three, Day Seven.

Follow the five steps carefully. *Record* your points for the day. Once more, reread the unedited statements taken from the recording (p. 55). CONGRATULATIONS!! You have now come to the end of WEEK THREE. If you accumulated *at least 500 points,* proceed to WEEK FOUR.

WEEK FOUR

Comments: "I had tried every known method of losing weight short of surgical invasion of my body. I just couldn't bring myself to that. This method of losing weight is to weight control what penicillin is to infection. It's revolutionary!" Those were the comments of Subject J-5 when she discovered that she was losing weight without being on a diet.

She had been on fad diets and lost weight. (Much of the weight that she lost while on those diets was probably glycogen and water and not fat.) When she went off the diets she regained the weight. When you reach your new weight you don't have to worry about what will happen when you "go off your diet" because you don't "go *on* a diet" to lose the weight in the first place.

You are now ready to begin WEEK FOUR of the program. Your subconscious or weight control center is probably already reset at the new level. Your weight is being adjusted downward. When your weight control center has completed its job, your waistline will again look the way it did when you were in high school or college. (If you are *now* in high school or college, it will look the way you think it *should* look for someone your age.) When your weight reaches a new, lower level, you will enjoy looking at yourself in the mirror. You will enjoy looking at photos of yourself.

There is another really good side to adjusting your weight downward. In addition to looking great, you are in the process of improving your health. Men who weigh 30 percent more than their ideal body weight have mortality rates that are 35 to 42 percent above normal! That is a *big* increase in mortality for being just 30 percent above your ideal body weight. It is a big price to pay. (It is fairly easy to get 30 percent above your ideal body weight if you put on a "middle-age spread.") Women who are 30 percent above their ideal body weight have mortality rates that are 25 to 30 percent above normal.

Obesity is associated with a lot of health problems. These problems—just to name a few—include high blood pressure, diabetes, gallstones, and higher levels of fat in the blood. As you can see, you are in the process of doing yourself a really big favor. You are in the process of looking better, feeling better, and making yourself healthier. *Congratulate yourself*!!

You are looking better, feeling better and making yourself healthier without subjecting yourself to the unpleasantness of unfamiliar food. You are eating the type of food that you have always been accustomed to eating. That's good! If you want a sandwich, eating all of the lettuce in central California isn't going to make you *not* want a sandwich.

Things to do during Week Four: It is important to concentrate on all five of the steps in the program. During WEEK FOUR give *special emphasis* to saying to yourself, "I'm full." This is an important step in the reprogramming process. Repeat the words "I'm full" to yourself whenever you think of eating, during the time you are eating, and whenever you think of this program. Write the words on a piece of paper and use the paper for a bookmark. In other words, any time it occurs to you to do so during WEEK FOUR, say to yourself, "I'm full." Make the words "I'm full" your motto. Let this be your special project for the week.

During WEEK FOUR follow the five steps just as you did during WEEK THREE. In addition, *each day of* WEEK FOUR repeat the following to yourself:

"It is very important that I remain focused on my goal. I realize that I have not lost all of the weight I want to lose but that is of no concern to me. That is the responsibility of my weight control center. It is not my duty to concentrate on losing weight at all. I am simply resetting the weight control center in my brain so that it can do the job that it is supposed to do. I must guard against focusing on weight loss and concentrate on resetting my weight control center. I must guard against becoming lax in my efforts at this point in time. It is particularly important that I concentrate on resetting my appestat at this time."

KEEPING SCORE DURING THE REMAINING WEEKS

Beginning with WEEK FOUR, the method of keeping score will be changed. You can now very rapidly mentally calculate your daily point totals. At the end of the day, you know whether you have accumulated 50, 75 or 100 points. You have been able to do this for some time but the *act* of keeping the score—the repetition—was necessary to help permanently change the nerve circuits. Keeping score adds to the repetition and indicates your degree of commitment. However, if you are unable to continue to write down your score, don't abandon the method.

At least, continue to mentally add up your score at the end of each day. If you wish to record the score—and this will reinforce the repetition—you may do it in a different fashion. You can simply write down one number, the *daily total*.

Obtain a spiral notebook, tablet or diary. Write the date at the top of the page. On the left side of the page, write DAY 1, DAY 2, etc. (see below). Leave enough space so that you can make a comment about your thoughts or activities. This will provide a permanent record for you. When you record your comments daily (if you wish to do so), and keep a daily score, you will be providing some much-needed repetition to the nerve circuits that you are retraining. At the end of DAY 7, tally your points for the week and record them just as you did during the first three weeks.

Your keeping score in this fashion is optional. The Appestat Program will work even if you don't record the points.

Below is an example of this type of scorekeeping:

DAY 1: Comment: *"Walked for 15 minutes."*

_____Daily Total: *100*

DAY 2: Comment: *"Noticed that I no longer have the craving for chocolate; walked a mile."*   Daily Total: *100*

Be sure to include your "comments." Give yourself the proper number of points for each day and record them beside "Daily Total." Add 10 points to the total for each day if you record your points on the day you follow the steps. Subtract 10 points if you record them at a later date.

(We have evidence to indicate that the rate of weight loss is *directly proportional* to the daily accumulation of points.)

You have come to the end of the first four weeks of the program. Weigh yourself.

WEIGHT AT THE END OF WEEK FOUR:_____

If your weight control center has adjusted your weight downward by two to four pounds, you have done an excellent job of following the steps. *If your appestat has adjusted your weight downward by more than four (4) pounds, check your food intake to be certain that you are getting a balanced diet.* There are a number of nutrition source books. You might wish to consult one of them and your physician for information. The following is an example of a source of helpful information on nutrition: Food and Nutrition Board, *Recommended Dietary Allowances* (9th rev. ed.). Washington, D.C.: National Academy of Sciences, National Research Council, 1980).

WEEK FIVE

Comments: Before beginning WEEK FIVE, stop for a moment to consider the term "obesity". (Comments regarding the term "morbid obesity" appear next week). "Obesity" is nothing more than an accumulation of too much fatty tissue. A person is considered to be obese when he or she is 20 percent above his or her ideal body weight. Some common sense should be used if you apply this definition of obesity to yourself. For example, a muscular athlete may be 20 percent above his ideal body weight and have very little fatty tissue. Conversely, an older person might have an accumulation of body fat and be only 10 to 15 percent above his ideal body weight.

Most people are not well-trained, muscular athletes. Consequently, if they have a body weight that is 20 percent above their ideal body weight, they probably have more fatty tissue than they need. Since you are five weeks into this program, you know it is easy to reduce the amount of fatty tissue that you do not want or need.

It is important to keep in mind that you want to lose weight by reducing the amount of *fatty tissue* in your body. You do not want to lose weight by depleting your body of water and glycogen—a valuable source of energy. For that reason you want to lose weight gradually.

To date, individuals who have lost weight by reprogramming their appestats have lost it at an *average* rate of 1.1 pounds per week. A weight loss of one-half to one pound per week is just about ideal. Although weight loss might average one-half to one pound per week over a period of many weeks, individuals typically lose weight in a stair-step fashion. That is, there is a decrease in weight, then a plateau which is followed by another decrease. (See Figure 2.)

Do not be afraid of the plateaus. They are temporary. Just concentrate on the steps that you are to follow. Over the long run your weight will gradually move to a new, lower level. It will do so at a rate that will allow your body metabolism to

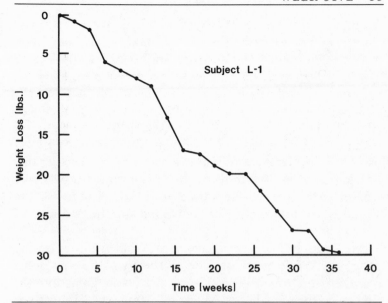

Figure 2. The change in weight of Subject L-1 is shown. Note the "stair-step" effect. Initially the subject lost weight, then there was a plateau which was followed by additional weight loss. Note also that the average weight loss was approximately one pound per week.

adjust, and at a rate that will allow for a reduction in the amount of *fatty tissue* in your body. If, during a plateau, your subconscious says, "It's not going to work for you," just say to your subconscious, "Oh *yes it is!* It has worked for everyone else! It not only *can* work for me, it *is now* working for me!" A few strong inputs of that message will take care of your subconscious.

Your subconscious, or appestat, is resetting your body weight to a new, lower level. You are looking better and feeling better. You are probably becoming more active. (More will be said later on the effect of weight loss on desire for increased physical activity!) You can take comfort in the fact that as you reduce the fatty tissue that you don't need, there is an improvement in the medical problems which accompany being overweight. Further, you reduce the risk of encountering other medical problems associated with "obesity."

Things to do during Week Five: Think about what you want. The body expresses what the mind dwells upon. This was brought home to me in a very surprising way during the course of a conversation I had with a friend of mine. He has a youthfulness and vitality that is inspiring. He is physically capable of doing more than most men, regardless of their age. Although he is well past 30 years of age, he has a strength and endurance that surpasses that of many 30-year olds. His unusual intelligence seems to improve with time. I suspected that he had passed his 50th birthday, but imagine my astonishment when I discovered that he was 69 years old! I had to ask him about it. He told me about something that he had learned early in life.

As a youth he had participated in the Golden Gloves boxing program. While working out at the gym, he saw some wrestlers—huge men—doing warm-ups before going into the ring to do their act. He asked one of them how he came to be so strong. The wrestler said, "If you stay around strong people, you'll get strong." That made a lasting impression on my friend. He remembers it to this day. He extended the reasoning. If it is true, he thought, that you will get strong by staying around strong people, maybe if you stay around young people—young in thought, not necessarily in chronological age—you will become young; if you stay around intelligent people, you will become intelligent; if you stay around happy people, you will become happy, etc. . . . He learned that the body tends to become what the mind is exposed to and dwells upon.

Your subconscious doesn't know what is real and what isn't. It only knows what you tell it. That's the reason you can reprogram it. If you tell it that you are a good athlete, a happy person, that you weigh ____ pounds or any other of a number of things, it accepts that as a fact and tends to have you become that type of person. Perhaps you have heard that "you become what you think." That's an old saying, but old sayings get to be old for a reason: there's usually some truth to them.

Tell yourself that you are trim. Don't *allow* yourself to think of yourself as being any way other than as trim and as physically fit as you wish to be. Remember, the body expresses what the mind dwells upon.

Remind yourself that *moderation is important*. Tell yourself that you are attracted to the idea of moderation in living, including dietary moderation.

Concentrate on all five of the steps *each day* during WEEK FIVE. Again this week give *special emphasis to saying to yourself, "I'm full." Read something from this book before every meal.* Even if you just pick it up, flip it open to a random page and read that page, you are sending a clear message to your weight control center that you still intend to have your weight controlled at a new level.

WEEK SIX

Comments: Individuals are considered to have "morbid obesity" if they are 100 percent above their ideal body weight. If a person's ideal body weight is 120 pounds and he weighs 240 pounds or more, he is considered to have morbid obesity. Individuals are also considered to have morbid obesity if their body weight is 100 pounds above their ideal body weight.

It was noted earlier (WEEK FOUR) that men and women who are 30 percent above their ideal body weight have mortality rates that are 25 to 42 percent higher than normal. Mortality rates are *even greater* in morbid obesity. The rates may be as much as *12 times* normal in morbidly obese individuals.

Consider this review of 16 morbidly obese individuals (quoted from Wilkins and Levinsky, *Medicine,* 3rd ed., Little Brown and Co., Boston, 1983, p.31). The average body weight of the 16 people in the study was 811 pounds! Perhaps that sounds like an unbelievable figure, but remember, there apparently is no upper limit to the amount of weight a person can gain. The people in the study quoted above didn't live very long. The average age at the time of death was *35 years!* That's tragic in view of the fact that life expectancy is now more than 70 years and is moving toward 80 years.

Since obesity is associated with a lot of medical problems, its prevention is of considerable importance to public health. Almost everyone recognizes that. They know that maintaining a proper body weight makes them more healthy. That's one reason so many attempts have been made to "override" or "fool" the weight control center. Another reason is that people simply want to look good.

People whose weight is above normal are at the mercy of their appestats. In order to lose weight and keep it off permanently, they are faced with having to override or fool their appestats for the rest of their lives.

Now that *your* weight control center has a new target, it can reset your body weight to a new level while you go about your business. Your weight will be reset. In the meantime you can feel "full." Visualize yourself at every moment as the trim person that you want to be.

In the "Introduction" it was pointed out that the appestat may be already set at birth. (Remember, it may be already set but the setting can be changed.) The fact that the appestat is already set at birth is probably the reason that identical twins who grow up apart from each other tend to have body weights that are similar to each other rather than body weights that are similar to their foster families. That is also the reason that different people have different body weights—their appestats are set at different levels. Most of us have known people who have been trim all of their lives, and people who have been 50 pounds overweight all of their lives. The weight of both remains constant from year to year. In both instances the appestat remains permanently set.

There is another type of person, the type who, at a certain time in life, begins to slowly gain weight. There are two reasons for this. First, individuals may start to slowly gain weight after reaching adulthood because the appestat remains set where it has always been set and the metabolic rate gradually decreases. The second reason individuals might start to slowly gain weight is slightly more complicated. It actually involves a gradual resetting of the appestat to higher and higher levels. How is this possible?

Animals—humans included—are able to store up some extra calories for emergency use. This is a protective mechanism which makes survival possible under adverse conditions. It is not necessary for the setting of the appestat to be changed in order for a few extra calories to be stored. The appestat likely plays a permissive role in allowing the animal to take aboard some extra calories, anticipating that the calories will soon be used. Usually they are. If the animal finds itself without food or is forced into a situation where increased physical activity is required, the stored calories are used. Over the long run the body weight of the animal is still maintained at the level set by the weight control center.

If the human animal doesn't find itself without food, or doesn't use the stored energy by being more active than normal, the body weight might stay at a level slightly higher than normal for a prolonged period of time. Only in the recent history of humans has this been possible. In earlier times it was a struggle for most humans just to get the required calories. These days it is possible for a large number of people to store extra calories on a regular basis. If the weight of a person stays slightly elevated for an extended period of time as a result of the storage of the extra calories, the appestat becomes less sensitive and probably gets reprogrammed to accept the new weight level as the norm. The appestat accepts the new weight level as its new setting. It will control the body weight at that level. If the individual doesn't eat, the appestat will send out "hunger" signals. Since the role of the appestat is to help insure the survival of the species, the signals can be very strong. If you have ever gained a few pounds during the holidays, then decided not to eat very much until those pounds disappeared, you have experienced those hunger signals. You know how strong they can be.

The only way to get the body weight to decrease permanently is to demonstrate to the appestat that it is going to be set at a lower level. That is what you are doing now as you follow the steps in this program. You are resetting it. If that is not done, the following cycle might develop—or continue: The appestat permits the body to take on a few extra calories, the calories are not used, the appestat readjusts its setting to a higher level, it again permits the body to take on a few extra calories, the calories are not used, the appestat readjusts its setting to a higher level, and on and on. The cycle repeats itself again and again. The body weight goes higher and higher.

As noted above, your appestat has a new target. It will reset your body weight to a new level. You only have the urge to eat if your appestat tells you that you do. For that reason, your body weight can be adjusted downward without your having to undertake the burdensome task of attempting to override the appestat.

By now you are probably getting the urge to become more physically active. That's okay. Don't suppress the urges. They are natural.

Things to do During Week Six: Concentrate on all five of the steps each day during WEEK SIX. *Record* your points *each day*. Remember that each step has its place in the reprogramming of your weight control center. Think about the words "I'm full" as often as possible. Remind yourself that moderation is important. On the first, third and fifth day of WEEK SIX reread the "comments." The *repetition* is important!

*Read **something** from this book before every meal!*

Chapter 4

Is There an Alternative To Obesity Surgery?
(Weeks 7–9)

WEEK SEVEN

Comments: I have heard people say, "I guess I'm just born to be fat." Maybe you have heard a similar expression. It is a tragedy to let people believe that they are "born to be fat" because it just isn't so. Maybe their ideal body weight *is* 115 pounds and they *weigh* 285 pounds. That doesn't matter. They are just as entitled to weigh 115 pounds as anyone else. They can. There is no law which says, "A trim waistline shall be reserved for a select few." Anyone who has set their appestat to a new level—to the level of their ideal body weight—will soon have their weight *controlled* at that level.

One individual (she has now *lost* 165 pounds!) said to this author, "I used to go into a store to buy clothes and ask 'where's the tent and awning section?' These days I buy the same stylish clothes as everyone else. It's a great feeling!" Today she weighs approximately 120 pounds. She was "cured" of being overweight. She was cured of her morbid obesity. What's more, *no drastic measures* such as surgery or hopitalization were required for her "cure."

"There's no 'cure' for me. I wouldn't lose weight if my jaws were wired together." Maybe you have heard that expression, too. Perhaps some of us have used the expression. You now know, of course, that once your weight control center does its job and sets your weight to the new level, you will be 'cured.' You won't have to think about such drastic measures.

Believe it or not, wiring a person's jaws together is one of the treatments which has been used to reduce body weight. As unpleasant as that procedure sounds, wiring the jaws together is the *least invasive* of the surgical techniques used to treat obesity. It does produce weight loss, but the weight loss *is not maintained* after the wire is removed. (You could have predicted that result based on the knowledge that you now have. It is virtually impossible to override the appestat permanently unless one is *forced* to do so.) The current feeling is that if this jaw-wiring procedure is used at all, it should only be considered as a means of preparing a morbidly obese person for obesity surgery.

Surgical procedures used to cure obesity will be discussed in coming weeks. Learning about obesity surgery impresses upon one the seriousness of the problem of obesity and underscores the difficulty which can be experienced by those who try to lose weight. Individuals with morbid obesity often resort to surgery only after all other avenues have been explored, only after all else has failed. Their appestat maintains their body weight at such a level that it is life-threatening. Still, losing even a few pounds seems an impossible task.

The person who is only ten to twenty pounds overweight likely experiences comparable difficulty in attempting to permanently rid himself of that amount of weight. In both situations—ten pounds overweight or morbidly obese—the individuals find themselves opposing their appestat. In both situations the appestat must be opposed or overridden for a lifetime. That is an enormous undertaking, whether it is attempted by an extremely heavy individual or by a mother who can't get rid of the extra 15 pounds she gained as a result of having two children. The appestat is indeed powerful. Its mission is to insure sufficient nutrient intake to sustain life. When viewed from that perspective, it comes as no surprise that attempts to override it have met with little success.

Several years ago while attending an international scientific conference, I met a bright woman scientist whose interest, like mine, was heart and blood vessel disease. She, as much as anyone (and more than most) knew of the deleterious effects of being overweight. She knew that being overweight enhanced heart and blood vessel disease, degenerative joint disease, diabetes and other diseases. Yet, she seemed to be completely at the mercy of her appestat.

She wore wide, flat, thick-soled shoes to help stabilize her as she walked. She waddled from side to side a bit as she made her way to the platform to speak. Her clothes, though expensive, were loosely draped over her body. They were cleverly designed to obscure, as much as possible, the extra weight she was carrying. Her scientific presentation was excellent. Following her lecture, she and I talked informally. Our discussion came around to the subject of the way the different control systems of the body keep variables such as blood pressure and heart rate regulated. We talked about how it is almost impossible to permanently change a variable in the body unless the setting of the control system is changed. We talked about some of the other control systems of the body. She mentioned that a person probably couldn't permanently change food intake and body weight unless he changed the *setting* of the control system which regulates them. I thought then (and am now convinced) that the setting of the food intake-weight control system (appestat) can be changed.

Two years later, I saw her at another scientific meeting, although—and I confessed this to her—I didn't recognize her at first. To begin with, she had lost more than 60 pounds of weight. In addition, she wore stylish high heels and fashionable clothes. She had new glasses, a new hairstyle and a spring in her step. She looked 20 years younger as she bounced up to the platform to speak. I was shocked! But the most shocking thing of all—and this I did *not* confess to her—was that when I first met her, I thought that she must be nearing retirement; that she must be at or near 60. She just had that "I'm getting old" look about her. Now, two years later, she looked like she was in her early 40s . . . as indeed she was! She, as always, gave an excellent scientific presentation. We again talked informally afterward.

I commented on the change which she had undergone. She told me that she had become determined to let her subconscious know that she was going to adopt a new lifestyle and that it might as well get used to the idea. Since that is what she was *expecting*, that is what she *got*. As far as I could tell from my conversation with her, she had not been on a diet. She had bombarded her subconscious over and over and over with the message that *it* was going to change; that she was going to be a different person. By doing so she apparently managed to reset her appestat. Then one thing led to another. When her weight decreased, she felt better, she looked better, she had more energy, she developed that spring to her step and a happier feeling about herself. She bought new clothes, got a new hairstyle, and became a new person.

You are doing the same thing that the scientist did. You are resetting your appestat. The difference is that you are resetting your appestat using a systematic method which has already been tested!

Continue to work on resetting your appestat. You are just as entitled to have the proper body weight as anyone else!!!

Things to do during Week Seven: Concentrate on all five of the steps each day during WEEK SEVEN. Record your points each day. Remember that each step has its place in the re-programming process. When you are on the way to breakfast, lunch or dinner say to yourself, "I'm full." Say the words, "I'm full" to yourself as you chew. Pause after the third bite of food, take a swallow of whatever you're having to drink, say to yourself, "I'm full," then continue to eat. When you have finished eating, get up from the table, pause and say to yourself, "I'm full." Constantly visualize yourself as looking the way you want to look.

Reread this week's comments at least twice during the week. Record your points *at the end of each day*. This provides more repetition than recording them all at once at the end of the week. Use the same type of recording system that you used for WEEK SIX. Include your comments when appropriate.

For additional repetition and reinforcement *read something from this book before every meal!*

WEEK EIGHT

Comments: Another 'cure' for morbid obesity is a surgical procedure which is commonly called "intestinal bypass." As the term implies, much of the digestive tract is "bypassed."

Normally the food that is swallowed goes from the stomach to the small intestine. It then goes to the large intestine. Anything which is not absorbed along the way is excreted. It is possible to surgically "bypass" most of the small intestine.

The small intestine is that part of the digestive tract where most of the food absorption takes place. For that reason, after the surgery, much of what one eats doesn't get absorbed and is excreted.

In the adult, the small intestine is approximately 20 to 22 feet long. It is divided into three parts; the first segment (the duodenum) is about one foot long. It is the upper segment of the small intestine and is attached to the stomach. The second segment (the jejunum) is about eight feet long. The third segment (the ileum) is approximately 12 feet long. It is attached to the large intestine.

The surgical procedure involves bypassing *most* (more than 15 feet!) of the second and third segments of the small intestine. Thus the procedure is called a "jejunal-ileal bypass." (See Figure 3.)

It probably doesn't surprise you that jejunal-ileal bypass surgery results in long-term weight reduction. Unfortunately, the weight reduction is often associated with some serious complications.

Following surgery, patients may have uncontrollable diarrhea, kidney stones, gallstones and other problems. They may become malnourished and have vitamin and mineral deficiencies. Strangely, most of the weight loss following this type of surgery is said to be a result of *decreased caloric intake*.

People with just a few pounds to lose aren't faced with deciding whether or not to have obesity surgery. In that respect they are fortunate. The decision must be an awesome

Intestinal Bypass Surgery

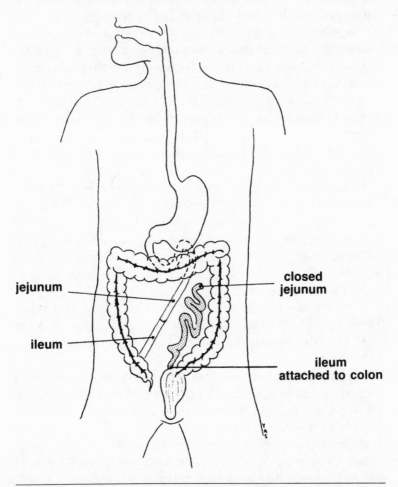

Figure 3. A segment of small intestine (shaded segment) has been disconnected from the digestive tract. The segment, which is more than 15 feet in length, is left attached to its blood supply and remains inside the body. One end of it is closed and the other end is attached to the colon. After surgery, anything that is swallowed goes from the stomach to the small intestine (jejunum and ileum), and then to the large intestine. The disconnected segment is bypassed.

one for those who face it. On the one hand there is the excess weight which threatens to reduce their life expectancy. On the other, there is the surgery with its possible attendant complications.

The fact that individuals are occasionally forced to have surgery for life-threatening obesity again underscores the difficulty one encounters when one attempts to *override* the weight control center for a lifetime. As mentioned earlier, it doesn't matter whether a person is trying to lose 150 pounds or 15 pounds, the level of difficulty is the same. In order for the weight to be kept off either individual *permanently,* the weight control center must be overriden *for the life of the individual*.

More about "cures" next week.

Things to do during Week Eight: Concentrate on *all five* of the steps each day during WEEK EIGHT. *Record* your points *each day*. Remember, the act of recording your score helps maintain your subconscious or weight control center at the new level.

Mental exercise in the form of visualization is an important part of the process of reprogramming the appestat. Do this new exercise *each day* of WEEK EIGHT: Close your eyes. Visualize yourself, at your new weight, wearing new, expensive clothes. Mentally examine every detail of your attire—the material, the color, and the accessory items. Really get a good picture of the way you look now that you have attained your ideal weight and are dressed this way. Visualize yourself as being a part of a happy occasion. After you have formed a clear mental image of your clothing and the occasion, *dwell* on the image for a while. Think of yourself as *being* in that situation. By doing so you are letting your appestat know the direction in which you are heading.

Read something—a line, a paragraph, or a page—from this book before each meal.

WEEK NINE

Comments: During the past few weeks you have been receiving information regarding "cures" for obesity. While you were assimilating that information, *your* body weight was decreasing—moving to a new, lower level. You now have an option for a "cure" which was not available when those procedures were being used. As your body weight continues on its way to the new level, consider some more "cures" for obesity.

The formation of a stomach "pouch" is the newest of the surgical procedures. (See Figure 4.) It involves surgically reducing the stomach from its normal size down to a small pouch capable of holding less than one-half cup. In addition to reducing the size of the stomach, the opening between the stomach and the small intestine is reduced to less than one-half of an inch. After this procedure has been performed, not much food can be put into the stomach. When food is put into the stomach, it can't leave the stomach very rapidly to enter the small intestine. Meal sizes must be drastically reduced. Individuals are *forced* to eat less than they normally would.

The procedure is not without complications. The pouch may develop perforations. Leaks may occur. It probably doesn't surprise you that patients may experience nausea and vomiting after they have had the surgery.

I was recently discussing the side effects of obesity surgery with a friend of mine whose specialty is family medicine. We were talking about how the lives of many morbidly obese people have been saved by surgery. He told me that he has had a few patients visit him following their surgery. They were no longer obese, but they came to him seeking medication to suppress their appetite. Because of their surgery they could only eat and absorb so much food but, unfortunately, they still *craved* food.

Methods other than surgery have been tried on individuals who are obese. One recent development is a device called the Garren-Edwards Gastric Bubble. It has been approved for use

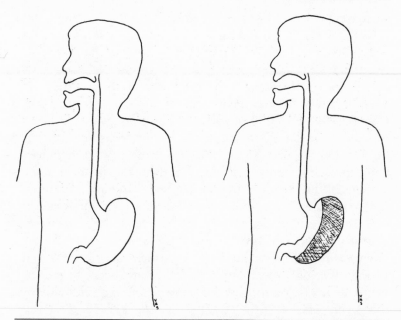

Figure 4. The effect of stomach stapling is shown. After surgery, a large part of the stomach (shaded area), can no longer hold or digest food.

by the FDA. The device is an inflatable cylinder which can be inserted through the mouth and into the stomach under light anesthesia. Once in place, the cylinder is inflated to a size of approximately two by three inches. Because it occupies space, it promotes a feeling of fullness. If, after several months, its size starts to decrease, it can be withdrawn and replaced by another bubble. The treatment may last eight to ten months. After that the bubble is withdrawn and the patient is allowed to rest for a few months.

The bubble results in a weight loss of one to three pounds a week. It was designed as a tool in weight loss and *claims are not made* that it is a *permanent cure* for obesity. It is recommended that patients undergoing treatment also receive counseling on nutrition and behavior modification.

Keeping weight off after it has been lost is a major problem with weight loss programs. Studies are being conducted in several universities to determine the long-term effectiveness on weight loss of the use of the bubble and concomitant supportive therapy.

A major disadvantage to the user of the bubble is the cost. The placement of the device plus follow-up visits can cost from $2,000 to $5,000 or more. A minor disadvantage is that it takes a few days for patients to become accustomed to the bubble. During that time they are likely to experience nausea and stomach cramps. Another disadvantage is the limited amount of time that the bubble can be left in place. There are other risks associated with its use, but they seem minimal.

As mentioned earlier, the bubble is meant to be a tool in the treatment of obesity, not a permanent cure for obesity. It does temporarily help individuals reduce their caloric intake. It appears that use of the bubble alone cannot serve to permanently control a person's weight, nor is that a claim made by the developers.

There are other types of "cures" for obesity. You could probably fill in the following blank with a *lot* of words. See if you can. Here is a phrase you have heard over and over again: "Have you heard about the _____ diet?" You *could* fill in the blank with a lot of words because you *have* heard about the "carbohydrate" diet, the "egg" diet, the "grapefruit" diet, the "tuna" diet, the "peanut butter" diet, the "protein" diet, the "liquid" diet and on, and on, and on. You also invariably hear that these diets are "really wonderful!," that so-and-so "lost 15 pounds the first week!" (Recall also, from earlier discussion, that diets which involve severe caloric restriction may cause an *increase* in body weight in the long run.)

A multitude of ingenious methods have been devised to help people fool their appestats. (Many of the methods also serve to "lighten" the person's wallet!) You know by now that a person's appestat can be fooled, but it can't be fooled *permanently*.

Fad diets are of no lasting benefit to individuals who use

them. Most of them may be harmless. One which is not deserves special mention. There are some diets of liquid protein derived from hydrolyzed collagen. Collagen is the major protein of the white fibers of connective tissue. When it is hydrolyzed, it is broken into simpler compounds, and there is an uptake of water molecules. Diets derived from hydrolyzed collagen have been associated with irregular heartbeats and death. They are dangerous! *They should be avoided!*

You are probably beginning to see a pattern emerge with respect to 'cures' for obesity. There are surgical procedures which *force* you to *override* your weight control center. There are a multitude of dietary manipulations which have been devised to help you *fool* your weight control center. Resetting the appestat appears to be a more physiologically acceptable solution.

Things to do during Week Nine: Use your imagination to reprogram your appestat. It can be done. An important psychological discovery of recent times was the discovery of the self-image. Everyone has an image of themselves. What they are and what they do depend on this self-image. If they want to change something about what they are or about what they do, then they can change their self-image. It has been proven time and again that if the image changes, the individual changes. If you tell yourself that you can't play tennis, if you have told yourself all of your life that you can't play tennis, if you have come to believe—to *know*—that your can't play tennis, do you know what? You're right. You *can't play tennis*. The reverse is also true. If you tell yourself that you can do something, if you come to believe it, to know it, then you very likely can do it.

How can the self-image be changed? By the vigorous use of your imagination, by the use of visualization, and by repetition. Albert Einstein thought that imagination was extremely important, that it was a revelation of things to come.

Imagination is important because your subconscious can't

tell the difference between experience and imagination. If you let your subconscious know enough times that you are trim, if you tell it that you are trim from now on, if you come to believe it—to *know* it—then your self-image changes. Once your self-image changes, it will become *necessary* for your subconscious to change your appestat in order to change *you* to fit the new image. When your self-image changes, you change. You can't help it!

Once your appestat is changed, it will keep you on target just as surely as a heat-seeking missile stays on target. If a heat-seeking missile strays to the left or right, or up or down, a correction will be made to bring it back on target. In a similar fashion, if your subconscious perceives you as weighing a certain amount, if it perceives you as trim, if it perceives you as being completely "full" at a reduced body weight, it will keep you on target.

Vigorously use your imagination, the visualization and the repetitious phrases to reprogram your appestat. Use the visualization of the ancient Greeks regarding dietary moderation. Eating was not a pastime with them. Tell yourself that eating isn't a pastime with you either.

Follow all five steps of the program. Again this week give special emphasis to saying "I'm full" whenever you think about the words.

Chapter 5

The "Energy-to-Burn" Feeling and the Cardiovascular System
(Weeks 10–14)

WEEK TEN

Comments: In the weeks that follow, some "miracle" cures for obesity will be examined. These "cures" are interesting in that they produce more health problems than they solve. The gadgets and diets which are on the market seem innumerable. Some try to help override the weight control center. Some try to help fool the weight control center. Some do neither and are outright fraudulent. The more popular ones will be discussed.

Before beginning WEEK TEN, it is important to have you examine and consider a subtle variation in your program for resetting your appestat. Physical exercise will be made an *optional* part of the program from this point on.

(Note: No one should undertake a program of exercise or increased activity without the advice of his or her physician.)

I believe that physical exercise contributes substantially to one's overall health. However, I wish to emphasize again that physical exercise is an *optional* part of this program. Even a person who is a paraplegic or one who has sustained mild to moderate paralysis as a result of a disease process can still use the program to reset his appestat. Now, having said that, I encourage you to make regular physical exercise a part of your daily routine.

What kind of exercise? Aerobic exercise is the best. By "aerobic exercise" I don't mean to imply that you need to join an aerobics class. (Exercise classes have borrowed the term "aerobics" because that is the type of exercise that they do.)

Here is the difference between aerobic exercise and ana-erobic exercise: If you run a 100-yard dash, that is an *anaerobic* exercise. While running, you use oxygen faster than you can breathe it into your body. When you finish running, you will breathe hard for a few minutes so you can "pay back" the oxygen that you used. If you walk or ride a bike around the block, you can breathe in oxygen at the same rate that you use it. When you do that you are doing an *aerobic* exercise. Walk-ing, bike-riding, tennis, and jogging are all examples of aero-bic exercise.

Exercise is an aid to good health. In addition, some experts believe that physical activity brings one's appetite into balance with his energy expenditure. Physical activity is not suggested here so that it will decrease your appetite. If it does decrease your appetite, it will probably do so without your being aware of it. You are not to be concerned about your appetite. That is the responsibility of your appestat. The option of physical activity is being added to the program because by the time individuals are this far along into the program, they typically comment that they feel "hyper" or "wired" or "have energy to burn." It is predictable that a person's energy level would increase. The increased activity which accompanies weight reduction has been observed in obese experimental animals. As their weight decreases, their level of activity increases sig-nificantly.

Have you ever heard people say, "He's skinny because he's so full of energy."? Maybe it's the other way around. Maybe they should say, "He's so full of energy because he's skinny." As time goes along, decide for yourself which of the two statements is correct.

There are some definite beneficial effects to be derived from increased activity. These will be considered during the coming weeks.

Q. I thought it was not necessary to engage in physical activity in order to reprogram the appestat.

A. It isn't. If you are comfortable following the five steps as you have been doing, you should continue to do so. The program will continue to work for you. The concept of activity is introduced as an option to those who are beginning to feel that they have more energy than usual—who feel good and want to burn some of that energy—who want that added 'bonus' of burning some extra calories. If you choose to continue the five steps you have been following, give yourself 100 points for each day you complete them. The program will continue to work.

The addition of activity to the program will alert your body to the fact that changes are taking place. It will also allow you to ease your "energy-to-burn" feeling. The activity you choose is strictly optional. You may choose to walk, walk while standing in place, wave your arms as if you were conducting an orchestra, rotate your upper torso from side to side, any combination of the above, or you may choose any other activity which you enjoy.

Whatever activity you choose, do it for 15 minutes each day. It doesn't have to be done continuously. You can do three five-minute periods of activity, five three-minute periods of activity, or even 15 one-minute periods of activity. It *is important* to remember that this physical activity is to be *in addition to* your normal daily routine.

Some of the scientifically demonstrated benefits of exercise will be detailed later. One good effect is that for every 15 minutes you spend doing a moderate exercise—walking, for example—you burn approximately 100 calories. That doesn't sound like much, but over a period of a year, that can reduce your body weight by ten pounds. A reduction in body weight of 50 pounds over a five-year period is a pretty good bonus for engaging in an activity that makes you feel better anyway. Don't substitute activity for the visualization and phrases. Make activity an addition to your program.

WEEK ELEVEN

Comments: It is difficult to hold back and not engage in physical activity when one feels "energized." Expending the pent-up "nervous" energy feels good.

When you exercise, you increase the amount of muscle tissue in your body. Because muscle tissue requires energy, the more muscle tissue you have, the more calories you will burn while at work, at play, or asleep in bed. Let's examine this further by describing two fictional characters.

John and Ted are both the same age and the same height. Both weigh 170 pounds and neither is overweight. John consumes 2800 calories a day to maintain his weight, while Ted can maintain his weight on 1800 calories a day. Here's why:

John needs more calories because only 12 percent (about 20 pounds) of his 170 pounds is fat. The remaining 150 pounds is *lean body mass*. Fat is a calorie storage depot, but the lean body mass consumes calories at a very rapid rate. Since John's 150 pounds of lean body mass is consuming calories around the clock, and because he burns an additional 300 calories each day by walking, he must consume 2800 calories a day to maintain his weight at 170 pounds.

Ted's situation is different. He weighs 170 pounds but approximately 30 percent (51 pounds) of his body weight is fat. He has only 119 pounds of lean body mass which will burn calories on a continuing basis (compared to John's 150 pounds of lean body mass.) In addition to having considerably less calorie-burning lean body mass, Ted doesn't burn additional calories by participating in an aerobic activity. For these reasons, even though he weighs 170 pounds, he can maintain his weight on 1800 calories a day. Should Ted decide to reduce his fat stores and increase his lean body mass by becoming more physically active, the increased physical activity will burn calories, and the additional lean body mass he will acquire as a result of the increased physical activity will burn calories. He will then have two options: He can continue to consume 1800 calories a day and *lose* weight, or he can *increase* his caloric intake and *maintain* his weight at 170 pounds.

Physical activity will increase your lean body mass. In addition, physical activity sends an important message to your appestat. When you become more active, your appestat gets messages from the "non-thinking" part of your nervous system. The "non-thinking" part of your nervous system lets your appestat know that your body needs to change. Your appestat gets information from the muscles that they are going to be alive with activity; it gets messages from the heart and blood vessels that the heart is going to pump more blood; and it gets messages from the temperature regulating system that the body is going to be perspiring and dissipating heat. In short, physical activity notifies the brain that the body needs to begin operating more efficiently; that it needs to change from an energy-storing machine into a "lean machine"; and that the ratio of lean body mass to body fat needs to increase. The brain gets the message that the body needs to "waste" some fat in order to become more trim.

The most important way to change your appestat is to bombard it with the "thinking" part of the brain by using the repetitious phrases and visualization outlined in this book. But when you become more physically active, you are also sending messages from the "non-thinking" part of your brain to your appestat. Those messages will help reset your appestat *and* increase the amount of calorie-burning, lean body mass in your body.

There are some scientifically proven positive benefits to physical activity. It has long been a popular belief that physical exercise might *increase life expectancy* as well as preserve some of the desirable qualities of life. Scientific evidence now supports those beliefs.

Exercise decreases body fat. People who initiate a program of exercise increase their ratio of lean tissue to fatty tissue. There is evidence that increased activity lowers the blood pressure, reduces the resting heart rate, and reduces the level of the harmful low-density lipoproteins (fat) in the blood. All of these changes which exercise brings on are associated with an increase in life expectancy.

That exercise does increase life expectancy was recently confirmed in an extensive, well-designed study of more than 16,000 men. The study extended over a period of 16 years (Paffenbarger, Hyde, Wing and Hsieh, 1986). The men were examined in relation to mortality from *all causes*.

Their exercise consisted of everything from regular walking to participation in sports. Death rates decreased steadily as energy expended on those activities increased. Death rates were one-fourth to one-third lower among those who expended an extra 2000 calories a week. (Remember, that was a lower death rate from *all* causes.) The older men at the highest level of activity had *half the risk* of those at the lowest level of activity! Younger men at the highest level of activity had 25 percent less risk than those at the lowest level of activity.

Scientists who have studied longevity have questioned whether it is possible to modify the *aging* process. The study of Paffenbarger and his group which was quoted above does not answer that question, but it does add evidence to support the view that physical exercise *increases life expectancy*.

Several interacting variables determine survival. Some are hazardous (high blood pressure, hardening of the arteries) and some are beneficial (proper diet, weight control, sufficient rest). Physical activity is a beneficial variable.

(Note: Some factors which may influence the *aging* process will be included in later discussions.)

Things to do during Week Eleven: Concentrate on all five of the steps. Remember to tell yourself that you are "slim and trim," that you "weigh _____ pounds." Think of yourself as trim. Remember to say to yourself "I'm full" whenever the words occur to you but especially when you are eating. Think about the ancient Greeks. Think about having a few green vegetables and some bread to eat. Think of eating as a necessary function rather than as a pastime, and concentrate on the quality of the food rather than the quantity.

WEEK TWELVE

Comments: Have you ever heard anyone make the following statement? "I only have so many heartbeats in my lifetime. I'm not going to use up any of them by exercising." A similar comment, which was made by a well-known individual, recently appeared in one of the national news magazines. It is one of those statements which seems to make sense the first time you hear it. But after you examine it carefully you realize that it is a contradictory statement. If the individual *really believed* the statement, he or she would be out there exercising every day.

Consider the following example: One participant in this study, Subject H-1, decided to include the activity component in his program of resetting his body weight to a lower level. Prior to beginning the program, his resting heart rate was 78 beats per minute. (Get out your calculator if you want to follow along on the arithmetic.) When his resting heart rate was 78 beats per minute, his heart was beating 4,680 times each hour ($60 \times 78 = 4,680$). Since there are 24 hours in a day, his heart was beating 112,320 times *each day* ($4,680 \times 24 = 112,320$).

It is remarkable to think that an individual's heart can beat more than 100,000 times a day, day in and day out, but it can. After H-1 was a few weeks into the body weight adjustment process, he started a program of exercise. His weight continued to decrease until it reached the level he had selected. He continues to exercise even though his weight is now set at the new level. He exercises approximately 120 minutes a week. Is he "using up" extra heartbeats by exercising? Let's analyze his current situation and see.

His resting heart rate is now 51 beats per minute. That means that his heart now beats 3,060 times each hour (instead of 4,680 times). It beats 73,440 times each day (instead of 112,320 times). H-1 exercises for a period of 30 minutes, four times a week. On those days his heart rate may increase by as much as 100 beats per minute during the 30 minutes that he is active. That's an extra 3,000 beats. If that 3,000 beats is added to the 73,440 normal beats, that brings his total number of heartbeats to 76,440 per day.

How has exercise affected the number of times H-1's heart beats each day? Before he started the program his heart rate was 112,320 beats per day. Now it is 76,440 beats per day. His heart now beats *35,800 fewer times each day!!*

Because of the reduction of his body weight and the increase in his physical activity, H-1 is *saving 35,880* heartbeats *per day.* Since he is saving 35,880 heartbeats per day, it is easy to calculate the number of heartbeats he is saving in one week or in one month. If you really want to see a shocking figure, multiply 35,880 by 365 to calculate the number of heartbeats he saves in *one year*!

If it is true, as some may believe, that individuals have only so many heartbeats in a lifetime, H-1 is much better off than he was before he began the program. Someone who says, "I have only so many heartbeats in my lifetime and I'm not gonig to waste them," will be out there doing exercises *if he believes his statement!*

Figure 5 shows the body weight, blood pressure, and heart rate of Subject H-1. As the body weight decreased, the blood pressure and the heart rate also decreased.

Things to do during Week Twelve: If you take up an activity that you enjoy, you may not be able to do as much of it as you would like to do at first. (Maybe you will only be able to ride the bike up and down the street a few yards and you would like to be able to ride it around the block several times.) Be patient. You will be able to increase your level of activity as time passes. Remember, 15 minutes each day is all you'll need to devote to activity. It can be mild activity and can be done in intervals (five three-minute intervals, three five-minute intervals or any other combination you choose).

Concentrate on *all* of the steps. Remember to say the words, "I'm full" to yourself whenever you think about them and especially when you are eating. Utilize all of your visuali-

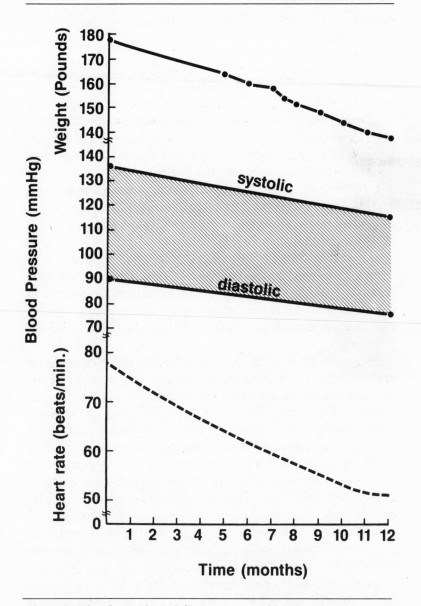

Figure 5. The change in weight (top curve), blood pressure (middle curve), and heart rate (lower curve) of Subject H-1 are shown. (See text for details).

zations. Remind yourself *each day* that you are saving some heartbeats.

WEEK THIRTEEN

Comments: Reducing your body weight and increasing your activity *will lower your blood pressure*. That's good! Hypertension—having a blood pressure that is higher than normal for a person's age—causes serious health problems.

Hypertension causes the heart to be enlarged. In later stages it may cause the heart or the kidneys to fail, or cause the individual to have a brain hemorrhage (stroke). High blood pressure injures the cells which line the inside of the blood vessels of the body. That damage increases the rate of development of atherosclerosis (hardening of the arteries) and may lead to a myocardial infarction (heart attack). Adults with blood pressure greater than 140/90 are considered to be hypertensive. They are treated to reduce the likelihood of complications.

Loss of body weight reduces the blood pressure. Aerobic exercise also reduces the blood pressure. If a person's blood pressure can be lowered with weight reduction and exercise, that is much better than treatment with drugs. That alone makes it worth the effort required to reset the appestat.

Here is an example of why nonmedical intervention such as weight loss is preferred in the treatment of hypertension: Diuretics are the most commonly used drugs for initial hypertension therapy. They are mild drugs, but they have side effects. They may cause you to lose potassium, cause you to have irregular heartbeats, cause muscle weakness, cause an elevation of blood sugar (or even diabetes), and cause the blood fat levels to increase. It is beyond the scope of this book to include a listing of the side effects of all of the drugs used to treat hypertension. The fact that drugs *have* side effects is mentioned to make the point that it is better to reduce the blood pressure without them *if possible*. If drugs are required to treat the hypertension, they should be used. There may or may not be side effects. Don't be tempted to leave off your high blood pressure medication if it is needed to control your hypertension. Uncontrolled hypertension damages the vital organs of the body.

The "Comments" of WEEK TWELVE concerned Subject H-1 and the number of heartbeats he saved each day as a result of his body weight adjustment program and his regular physical activity. The body weight adjustment program and regular physical activity had another very positive effect on Subject H-1. Prior to beginning the program his blood pressure was 138/90. He was a borderline hypertensive and probably would have been given drugs to control his blood pressure if it had not come down.

By the time his body weight had been set to a lower level—and his weekly physical activity had increased—his blood pressure had decreased from 138/90 down to 116/72. That is *well* within the normal range and reduces the possibility of complications he might have had if his blood pressure had remained high.

You are reducing your blood pressure now! As your body weight is being adjusted to a lower level, your blood pressure is *decreasing!*

Things to do during Week Thirteen: Follow *all* of the steps during WEEK THIRTEEN. Recording the points is an important part of the resetting process.

If you decided on aerobic exercise as a part of your program, you are probably finding, as someone put it, that "expending energy generates energy." That seems to be true. More about that and some words about the "addicting" effect of aerobic activity in coming weeks. For now, follow the steps and record your points.

WEEK FOURTEEN

Comments: If you can raise the level of the *HDL* in your blood, you can give yourself more protection against hardening of the arteries.

What is HDL? Lipids (fats) in the blood which are attached to proteins are called lipoproteins. Some of these complexes are heavier—have a higher density—than others. Consequently, they are called high-density lipoproteins (HDL). The ones with the lower density are called low-density lipoproteins (LDL). These are very important substances.

The *HDLs protect* against atherosclerosis. The *LDLs cause* atherosclerosis—hardening of the arteries—to develop at a faster rate. It follows then that if you want protection against atherosclerosis, you want the level of HDL in your blood to be high and the level of LDL in your blood to be low.

Is it possible to do something to raise the level of the good HDL in your blood? Yes. As a matter of fact you are *now* in the process of raising your blood HDL level.

Weight reduction is associated with high blood levels of HDL. (Conditions such as diabetes and obesity are associated with low blood levels of HDL.) Since you are in the process of reducing your body weight, the HDL levels in your blood are *increasing*. That will offer you added protection against the development of atherosclerosis.

The exact mechanism by which high blood levels of HDL protect against hardening of the arteries is not completely understood. It is known that if the cells which line the blood vessels are repeatedly injured, atherosclerosis progresses at a faster rate. It may be that HDL makes those lining cells stronger and more durable, or maybe the HDL protects them in some other fashion. Whatever the mechanism, maintaining high blood levels of HDL *is* protective against atherosclerosis. (Since *LDL* speeds the atherosclerotic process, it is possible that LDL makes the cells which line the blood vessels weaker and more fragile.)

You are also raising your blood HDL levels by being active.

Aerobic activity raises the blood HDL levels. Thus you are doing two things—lowering your body weight and engaging in aerobic activity—which will raise the HDL level in your blood.

Have you ever heard a statement similar to the following? "There's nothing you can do about hardening of the arteries. If you're going to get it, you're going to get it."? The statement is not correct. As a matter of fact, there are *several things* that people can do about atherosclerosis. They can raise the level of the desirable HDL in their blood by adjusting their body weight downward and by participating in aerobic activity. They can reduce the level of the harmful LDL in the blood by eating a proper diet—one containing less saturated fat and fewer cholesterol-containing foods. They can keep their hypertension under control.

Reducing blood cholesterol levels may be even more beneficial than previously thought. A recent study revealed that as little as a ten percent increase in blood cholesterol levels can result in a significant (29 percent or more) increase in the risk of dying from heart disease.

The study was done at 22 U.S. medical centers and included more than 350,000 men aged 35-57. The results, published in the *Journal of the American Medical Association,* (Stamler, 1986), show that even moderately elevated levels of cholesterol can markedly increase the risk of dying from heart disease. How much does the risk of dying from heart disease increase as the blood cholesterol levels go up?

In the study, the lowest death rates from heart disease occurred in men whose blood cholesterol levels were below 182 milligrams per deciliter (mg/dl) of blood. There was a *29 percent* increase in death rates from heart disease in those whose blood cholesterol levels were only slightly higher (182 to 202 mg/dl). Blood cholesterol levels above this were associated with much higher death rates from heart disease. If the blood cholesterol levels were 203 to 220 mg/dl, the death rates were *73 percent* higher than if they were below 182 mg/dl; if the blood cholesterol levels were 221 to 244 mg/dl, the death rates were *121 percent* higher than if they were below 182 mg/dl; and if the blood cholesterol levels were above 245 mg/dl, the death rates were *242 percent* higher than if they were below 182 mg/dl. The adverse effect of elevated blood cholesterol levels is worse than previously thought. In fact, death rates are elevated at blood cholesterol levels not previously considered dangerous.

The study clearly demonstrates that moderately raised levels of blood cholesterol can increase the risk of dying from heart disease. On the other hand, it is reassuring to learn that people can dramatically reduce their risk of death from heart disease by lowering their blood cholesterol levels only a few percent.

As you continue on this program of body weight adjustment, you are raising the level of HDL in your blood, lowering your blood pressure, reducing your heart rate, reducing your risk of heart failure and stroke, reducing your risk of coronary heart disease and a heart attack, looking and feeling better, and at the same time becoming energized. That's a pretty good bonus for a few months of patience and concentration!

(More next week on becoming energized.)

Things to do during Week Fourteen: The act of filling in the blanks with your score is an *important part* of the process of resetting your weight control center. It helps keep you on track; helps keep the momentum going in the direction you want it to go; and helps keep your target weight clearly in focus. As you go through the steps each day, as you remember to say to yourself, "I'm full" every time you think about it, as you participate in some type of aerobic activity, keep reminding yourself of all of the good things that you are doing *for* yourself.

Chapter 6

A Desirable "Addiction" and the Elimination of Stress
(Weeks 15–17)

WEEK FIFTEEN

Comments: Recent scientific findings have revealed a mechanism by which a person might become "addicted" to aerobic activity. (It's okay to become addicted. Remember the study of Paffenbarger and his group? The older men in the study who were at the highest level of physical activity had half the risk of death of those at the lowest level of physical activity. The younger men at the highest level of physical activity had 25 percent less risk of death than those at the lowest level of physical activity.) The addiction to physical activity is beneficial if it is not carried to extremes. If you are going to have an addiction, this is a good one to have.

How can something that causes you to sweat and expend energy be addictive? That question has a number of answers. The simple answer would be that aerobic activity increases the blood level of a substance that brings a pleasurable effect. In reality the situation is much more complex. Let's begin at the beginning:

Some 20 substances can be obtained from the juice of the opium poppy; morphine and codeine are among them. They can change an individual's mood and offer relief from pain. When synthetic drugs with similar actions were developed, they were referred to as "opioid" (opium-like) drugs.

Opioid drugs can produce emotional states of euphoria. Self-medication with them in an attempt to alleviate depression can lead to addiction.

A few years ago substances which have opioid activity were found to exist in the body. Since these natural substances do have opioid activity, they are referred to as "endorphins" (endogenous morphine). When individuals exercise, the blood level of one of these newly discovered substances, b-endorphin, increases. Additional investigation will probably show that the blood levels of other endogenous opioids also increase with exercise.

The increase in the amount of these opioid substances in the blood may serve to partially explain the "good feeling" that aerobic activity produces. That may be the reason that aerobic activity is "addicting" for some individuals.

It is not surprising that nature would have individuals feel good when they exercise. Building in a reward would keep them doing something that is good for them.

Things to do during Week Fifteen: Activity will elevate your mood. That's good. It's also natural. Don't hesitate to try it if you feel the urge.

Perhaps you think you are too old to engage in some type of physical activity. Can you get too old to exercise? I don't know. You'll have to decide that for yourself. Today I talked to a gentleman who still exercises. He walks as he goes about his daily routine of doing things. Then every afternoon he spends about 20 minutes walking in his neighborhood. What is so spectacular about that? The thing that is different—not necessarily spectacular—about that is that he celebrated his 100th birthday on February 11, 1987. Mr. Albert Sidney Carl of Jackson, Mississippi, was born during the time Grover Cleveland was President of the United States. He has lived during the terms of Presidents Cleveland, Harrison, Cleveland (second term), McKinley, Theodore Roosevelt, Taft, Wilson, Harding, Coolidge, Hoover, Franklin Roosevelt, Truman, Eisenhower, Kennedy, Johnson, Nixon, Ford, Carter and Reagan.

Mr. Carl's mother was a young girl during the Civil War. His grandfather, who died during the Civil War, had served under General Albert Sidney Johnston (thus the origin of Mr. Carl's name.)

Mr. Carl remembers the first automobile that he ever saw (a Maxwell) and remembers seeing steam cars. He remembers watching workmen string telephone lines from Memphis to New Orleans. He went to work for the telephone company as a messenger boy at the age of 12 and has been busy since. He still has busy days. After breakfast he might still go into his shop to work on one of the electrical appliances he takes apart and puts back together.

He told me that he has never been overweight, that he has never been the type to overeat and that he can still eat whatever he wants. He is just as bright and alert as ever. His daughter, a young 81-year-old, says that he might be in better shape now than he was when he was 60 years old. He is certainly erect and his eyes still shine with energy. He has seen a lot of changes during his lifetime but said he had never worried about what might happen. He always had so much to do, he didn't have time to worry. Even so, he said that he never felt stressed or felt that he had to "keep up with the Joneses."

Mr. Carl doesn't look, act or think "old." He admitted to me that he doesn't feel old.

Obviously he doesn't think he is too old to be active. If you are older than he is, you'll have to decide for yourself whether or not you're too old to engage in some type of physical activity. If you are younger than he is, it is probably okay for you to do so.

Remember that *all* of the steps in the body weight adjustment program are important. If you participate in an activity, during the time you are active, *visualize* yourself as being at your new weight.

WEEK SIXTEEN

Comments: *You have reached a milestone!!* Since you have

completed 15 weeks of the body weight adjustment program you have an understanding of what it takes to reset your weight control center to a new level. You will have absolutely no problem in carrying your program to its completion.

You will find the following questions and answers interesting. The subject was a participant in this program. You can probably relate to many of the feelings the subject experienced.

Q. How do you feel?

Subject: Fine.

Q. You look like you've lost some weight. Have you?

Subject: Yes. I've lost a lot. Now I weigh exactly what I weighed the day I graduated from high school.

Q. Did you ever think you would weigh that again?

Subject: No.

Q. Have you ever lost weight before?

Subject: Yes.

Q. What happened?

Subject: I gained it back.

Q. Are you gaining any of it back now?

Subject: Not a pound.

Q. Has anything else changed?

Subject: I'm more active.

Q. You look like you're in pretty good physical condition. Are you?

Subject: Better than I was.

Q. Do you do a lot of exercise?

Subject: No, not too much.

Q. What kind of exercise do you do?

Subject: I run. I do sit-ups and push-ups.

Q. How much do you run?

Subject: I do a 30-minute run, five times a week.

Q. How fast do you run?

Subject: Ordinarily I jog slowly but lately I've found myself running fast—almost sprinting—off and on during my runs. I just like the feel of running fast.

Q. How many sit-ups do you do?

Subject: Two hundred a day.

Q. *Two hundred!!*

Subject: Not all at one time! I do 20 at a time, ten times a day.

Q. That's still a lot. Doesn't it take a lot of time?

Subject: No. I do some in the morning before I go to work. I do a few during the day when there is no one in my office. I do a few in the evenings. I can do 20 sit-ups in 45 seconds. I do that ten times a day.

Q. Do you do bent-knee sit-ups?

Subject: Yes. I sit on the floor with my toes under something and do them.

Q. And the push-ups?

Subject: I do 20 at a time, five times a day.

Q. You do 100 push-ups a day!

Subject: Yes.

Q. When you began exercising, how much did you do?

Subject: I started out doing five sit-ups every other day and three push-ups a day.

Q. And the running?

Subject: At first I'd walk a few steps, then trot a few. I'd do that for a few minutes then stop.

Q. Do you plan to continue doing the exercises?

Subject: Oh, definitely. Exercise makes me feel good. I couldn't think of not doing it.

Q. Did you ever strain yourself or hurt yourself when you first started your program of exercise?

Subject: No. I made it a point not to overdo it.

Q. Have you been checked by a physician?

Subject: Yes. A cardiologist checked out my heart and tested me on a treadmill.

Q. You checked out okay?

Subject: Yes.

Q. What do you consider the most effective part of this body weight adjustment program?

Subject: I can see that all of the steps are important but two things helped me a lot. Saying "I'm full" helped and the activity part of the program made me feel good.

Q. Do you go hungry?

Subject: No.

Q. Never?

Subject: Never.

The individual above is doing more exercise than is required for cardiovascular fitness. It is clear from his answers that he is exercising more than necessary because of the 'good feeling' he gets from it.

Things to do during Week Sixteen: You can reset your body weight to a new level without exercising at all if you wish. If you do choose to include exercise as a part of your program, do something that you enjoy and take a sensible approach to it. Continue to constantly utilize the phrases and the visualizations.

WEEK SEVENTEEN

Comments: The comments of last week dealt with a subject who exercised because of the "good feeling" which resulted from the activity. It has been reported that exercise can produce a "high." States of "euphoria" have been described by individuals who engage in prolonged physical activity. Some of the opioids which the body produces (b-endorphins and probably other endorphins) do increase with physical activity, but whether they are entirely responsible for the feelings of euphoria is still open to question. They probably do contribute to it but there are likely other contributing factors as well.

Exercise can produce positive moods in individuals. Increased blood endorphin levels may be partially responsible. And furthermore, it will be difficult for you to have negative feelings about yourself when you are doing something so positive for yourself—doing something that is so good for you. Because of the accumulated evidence regarding the development of a positive mood with exercise, exercise programs have been recommended for the treatment of depressive illness.

Exercise can increase a person's tolerance to pain. That's not too surprising. It would seem reasonable that the "opioids" produced by the body would make a person less sensitive to pain just as morphine or synthetic "opioids" would make a person less sensitive to pain. Maybe this adds to the "addicting" effect.

The subject mentioned last week who runs for 30 minutes five times a week, then does 200 sit-ups and 100 push-ups each day would seem to be 'addicted' to activity. That is a lot of additional activity for anyone to incorporate into his daily routine regardless of his age. (The subject in question is more than 50 years "young"!) It is interesting that when he was asked whether he did a lot of exercise he said, "No, not too much." He didn't realize that he was actually doing quite a lot of exercise.

If something brings pleasure, produces euphoria or a "high," if repeated exposure is required for the pleasure or euphoria to continue, if withdrawal signs appear upon discontinuation, then that "something" can be said to be "addicting." Aerobic activity fits that description.

Scientists have found it difficult to study the effects of discontinuing aerobic activity. Individuals who do a significant amount of aerobic exercise are reluctant to stop for a period of time to be studied, even if they are paid to do so. Individuals who are forced to stop exercising because of an injury often experience changes in sleep patterns, become anxious, tense, and irritable. In other words, they have withdrawal symptoms.

You need not be reluctant to start a program of aerobic activity because you are afraid it will become a burden. It won't. It will actually lighten your mood. Nature has seen to it that you will be rewarded for exercising.

Again, remember that walking is a good aerobic activity. Recall also that a 15-minute walk each day burns enough calories to result in a 10 to 12 pound weight loss in 12 months.

Aerobic activity will help you feel less stressed. Few things will make you look younger, feel younger, be healthier, and live longer than *eliminating the effects of stress on your body*. By reducing your body weight, you are eliminating the effects of stress on virtually every system in your body. Certainly your cardiovascular, digestive, endocrine and respiratory systems will fare better as a result of the weight reduction.

Removing other types of stress, particularly mental stress, will actually enhance your weight reduction and contribute to the health and well-being of all of the different systems of your body. How can you eliminate stress? In a word, practice! Let us examine the process of stress and the effects it has on the body before we discuss ways to eliminate it.

Years ago, Dr. Hans Selye developed a unifying concept of stress when he noted that the body responded the same way to a wide variety of stimuli (Selye, H., *The Stress of Life,* New York, McGraw-Hill Book Co.). He described stress as being produced by diverse noxious agents and named the agents that produce stress, "stressors."

Stressors are usually extreme stimuli. If we have been accustomed to comfortable surroundings and casual company, we may be stressed by extreme heat, by extreme cold, by being in a large crowd or by being alone. Stressors may be unpleasant or painful but not always. A roller coaster ride might be fun and painless and still "stress" an individual because of the excitement.

It's also a fact that we don't all respond to stressors the same way. If a gregarious comedian and an introverted scientist were forced to change places, both would likely be stressed. Thus a stimulus that is a stressor to one person might not be a stressor to another.

Not all stressors are physical stimuli. Psychological stimuli stress individuals as much as, or more than, physical stimuli. An individual might be stressed by something that he or she *perceives* as a threat. The threat need not be real. A person may be stressed if he *thinks* something is a threat to either his survival or his self-image. Stress may be chronic or acute.

There are all kinds of acute, perceived threats which stress individuals. Here is an example: You hear a noise in your house late at night. You are alone. Your heart rate increases, the blood vessels supplying blood to your skin and intestines constrict and shunt the blood to your muscles. Rapid, small muscular contractions cause you to tremble. Your blood pressure goes up. Your heart pounds. You hear the noise again! There is a tightening-up of the muscles in your intestine. Your adrenal glands—small glands which are near your kidneys—pour adrenalin into your blood stream. Your heart pounds even harder; your mouth is dry; you are breathing rapid, shallow breaths; your palms sweat. You are experiencing the "fight or flight" reaction. Then you discover that your cat made the noise by turning over the sewing box. The threat was not real. After a few minutes all of your systems are back to normal. You breathe a sigh of relief. The threat was perceived, but the physiological responses were *exactly the same* as if it had been real! We react mildly or strongly to real and perceived threats every day. Repeated reactions to too much stress can adversely affect us and have a negative effect on our health.

We experience stress many times during our lifetime. Most of the time we adapt. Most of us experience stress of some type every day. We may be temporarily "alarmed" but we usually cope with it. We may be stressed if we fear something. That is good if it keeps us from driving too fast on a wet street. It is not good if it keeps us from achieving a goal—"I'm afraid to try. I might fail."

In addition to anxiety which can produce the "fight or flight" reaction, and fear which may inhibit or protect us, there are other types of psychological stressors. Among them are anger, worry, guilt, depression, poor self-image, and hate. In the interest of maintaining our physical and mental health, we need to eliminate those stressors. Those are chronic stressors which act on us over long periods of time to produce some predictable changes in our body. (See Figure 6.)

Chronic stress can trigger many diverse changes in the body. It does this by stimulating the hypothalamus to release a hormone called "corticotropin-releasing factor" or CRF. (Recall from earlier discussions that the hypothalamus is on the underside of the brain.) Chronic stress can also cause the release of adrenalin into the blood stream from the adrenal glands. This combination of responses to stress has diverse effects on the body.

Any factor which causes the release of CRF from the hypothalamus can initiate the changes. Usually these factors, these stressors, are injurious or extreme stimuli. The hypothalamus may be directly stimulated by injurious or extreme stimuli, or it may be indirectly stimulated in another way. Certain emotions such as worry or fear from the "thinking" part of the brain (the cerebral cortex) send stimulating impulses to the hypothalamus. These impulses can cause the hypothalamus to release CRF. In other words, an extreme physical stimulus or an extreme mental stimulus can cause the hypothalamus to release the same hormone.

The CRF, through a series of steps, causes another hormone, cortisol, to be released into the blood stream. The cortisol causes a decrease in the number of certain types of white blood cells. This results in a decrease in the immune response and a decrease in the allergic response. It also causes the breakdown of complex, stored sugars and elevates the blood sugar level. It increases the breakdown of tissue proteins. As a result of all of these changes, the ability to fight diseases, allergies, and infections is compromised.

Our goal is not to eliminate the stress reaction. Our reaction to stress is a mechanism which allows us to adapt to new situations. We want our bodies to react to stress only when necessary. What we don't want to do is set off the stress reaction when it is *not necessary*. Our goal is not even to eliminate all stress. Only the deceased are completely free of stress. We want to eliminate the *unnecessary* stress—especially eliminate the adverse effects of prolonged unnecessary stress

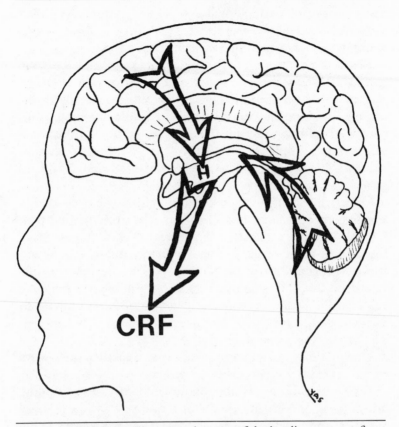

CRF

Figure 6. This figure illustrates that stressful stimuli may come from the "thinking" part of the brain (upper arrow). These stimuli may be in the form of emotions such as worry or fear. Stressful stimuli may also come from the "non-thinking" part of the brain (lower arrow) in the form of sensations such as pain or extreme temperatures. All of the stimuli are capable of setting off the stress reaction by causing the release of corticotropin-releasing factor (CRF).

which makes us more vulnerable to disease and which probably serves to speed the aging process.

Things to do during Week Seventeen. As you participate in an aerobic activity, *visualize* yourself as being at your new weight. (You become what you think!) Put that image of your new self in your mind so it will give your weight control center a clear target. Follow all of the steps as you have been doing. *Record* your comments and points in your notebook.

Take some positive steps to eliminate, avoid, or change your reaction to the stressors which you encounter daily. Aerobic activity will go a long way toward helping you change your response to stressors. Some other suggestions for eliminating mental stressors are given below. The suggestions are *examples* of ways to eliminate or change your reaction to certain stressors. They are given to illustrate that mental as well as physical stressors can be eliminated.

Ordinarily if an animal—the human animal included—is stressed, the animal adapts. If the stress is excessive and prolonged, a state of exhaustion can develop. When that happens, the adrenal glands enlarge, the lymphatic organs shrink, and stomach and intestinal ulcers develop. The resistance to disease decreases. The immune response is inhibited. An animal can actually die of excessive and prolonged stress. Individuals aren't usually stressed to that degree, but it is obvious that excessive stress is harmful.

During this week and during all of the weeks to come, work on getting rid of the following stressors.

Worry. You can worry about your children, house, car, dog, and clothes; or you can worry about the economy, the political situation and the threat of an ice age. (If you really want a long list of things to worry about, see Dyer, p. 117.) You can worry about an infinite number of things, but ask yourself the question, "What does worry accomplish?" You'll be surprised at your answer. Suppose you spend ten hours worrying because the United States became involved in World War II, or Vietnam. What would change? Nothing! The country was still involved and all of the destruction still occurred. Similarly if you worry about the weather being cold, or hot, or wet, or dry, if you worry that tomorrow is Monday, or if you worry that time is passing, all of those things are *still* going to happen. It's still going to be Monday, the weather is still going to be whatever it's going to be, and time is still going to pass no matter how much you worry. The same is probably true of the zillion other things that you can find to worry about. So why cause your hypothalamus to initiate the stress reaction over something that isn't going to change anway?

Try an experiment. Think of something, anything, to worry about. Worry about it for ten seconds—it could be ten minutes or ten hours, the result would be the same. Really concentrate and worry hard for ten seconds . . . Now, what changed? Nothing! If you *must* worry, set aside ten seconds every day, worry hard, and then be done with it until the next day when you again worry for ten seconds. That will take a great deal of stress off of you. Reducing stress will probably *significantly* assist your weight control center in reducing your body weight.

Fear. Fear is usually one side of a coin. The other side is *confidence.* Change "I'm afraid I can't" to "I'm confident that I can." Change, "I'm afraid I can't find time for some aerobic activity" to "I'm confident that daily aerobic activity will make me feel good." Change, "I'm afraid that my job will stress me today" to "I'm confident that I can handle things."

Having confidence will increase the odds that things will happen the way you want them to happen. Developing confidence will help you be in control of situations instead of letting situations control you. If you feel like you have to fear something, limit the amount of time during your day that you allot to it. During the other times *practice* thinking, "I'm confident that . . ."

A wise man once said, "I'm old now and I've had a lot of troubles, most of which never happened." That's the way many of our fears turn out.

Anger. Anger perhaps seems a natural reaction to some situations. That may or may not be true. It is true that some individuals have found it possible to control excessive anger by telling themselves that they are going to delay getting angry— count to ten or wait 30 seconds—when the situation arises. Once they are able to delay it for a few seconds, they attempt to delay it for longer and longer periods as other situations arise. I met one individual who was able to rid himself of frequent, uncontrolled outbursts by asking himself the question, "Do I really *care* enough about what he/she thinks, says, or does to let myself get angry over it?"

Perhaps anger, even feigned anger, is natural, and maybe it sometimes seems necessary. But one might ask the following questions: Is getting angry worth the effects it has on *my* body? Is it worth having CRF and adrenalin dumped into *my* system? Is it worth the effect it has on my adrenal glands, on my lymph organs, on my heart and blood vessels and on my white blood cells? If it isn't, then maybe it isn't worth getting angry.

Hate and *Revenge*. Why allow someone or something that you dislike to initiate the stress reaction in you and injure *your* health—maybe even shorten *your* life? Why allow that person to exert that influence over you? There is an old saying that "Time wounds all heels." Maybe it does, or maybe with time all heels wound themselves. In any event, why let something or someone wound *you*? You can help prevent it by working to eliminate two chronic stressors: hate and revenge.

Guilt. So you did something that you shouldn't have done? You also neglected to do something that you should have done? You led someone to believe something that wasn't true? You said something to someone that you shouldn't have said? You neglected to say something to someone when you should have or when you had the opportunity to? Okay, so what else is new? Who *hasn't* done those things at one time or another during his lifetime? Most people realize that those are very human things to do; they don't continue to punish themselves for having done them.

If you insist on feeling guilty, try the same thing that you tried with worry. Think of something that you really want to feel guilty about. Now try to feel just as guilty as you possibly can for ten seconds. (There is no point in feeling guilty for a longer period of time when you can accomplish just as much by feeling guilty for ten seconds.) What changed after you felt guilty for ten seconds? Nothing!

Is your feeling guilty worth causing your hypothalamus to initiate the stress reaction? Is your feeling guilty worth affecting your health when it isn't going to change things anyway? If you are one of those types who thinks that you will "just have to feel a little guilty sometimes," limit it to ten seconds a day. That will free up the rest of the day for more productive endeavors.

Depression. Aerobic activity is a good antidote for depression. Try it! It won't be easy to feel depressed while you are engaging in an activity that is so good for you. Many people have found that it is important to do *something* when they feel depression start to creep in on them. And doing something might be the key to combating depression. Doing what? Writing a letter, planting a flower, going for a walk, talking to an old person, helping a child, listening to some upbeat music, talking to or visiting someone who is enthusiastic about life, making a list of things to do if you ever start to feel depressed again—the list could go on and on. It will be difficult for you to feel depressed *and* do things at the same time.

There is another good reason for doing things. Someone once said that it is important to go, see, do and experience things because you are "such a short time alive and such a long time dead." So get up and get going!

The above are some emotions that can originate in your cerebral cortex, the "thinking" part of your brain. When the emotions originate in the cortex, impulses go from the cortex to the hypothalamus and initiate the stress reaction. As you work at eliminating both physical and mental stress, you are freeing up your mental and physical resources for more productive things.

Until you are able to prevent one or more of the above stressors from affecting you, try this: Set aside ten seconds each day to have the emotions. Determine that you will worry, be afraid, feel guilty, whatever, *only during that time* and that at no other time will you allow the emotions to stress you. Should any of the thoughts try to creep into your thinking, remind yourself that you will deal with them the next day at the appointed time. (Then each day cut back on the amount of time that you spend on them!) If you spend ten seconds dealing with these stressors, that will leave the remaining 23 hours, 59 minutes and 50 seconds for you to feel a relief and a freedom to fully enjoy your day! It will take *practice*, but you can do it!

Chapter 7

Control Systems and Getting "Old"
(Weeks 18–20)

WEEK EIGHTEEN

Comments: If your body temperature rises above 98 degrees, you will start to sweat. The sweat will evaporate and cool you. Your temperature will be lowered back to 98 degrees. If your body temperature falls below 98 degrees, you will start to shiver and maybe put on some warm clothes. That will raise your temperature back up to 98 degrees. Your body temperature is controlled automatically.

The amount of fluid in your body is controlled automatically. If you lose fluid, you will get thirsty and drink. If you drink too much fluid, your kidneys will eliminate the excess.

If you exert yourself for a few seconds and need more oxygen, you will breathe faster without even thinking about it. When you sleep at night and need less oxygen, you breathe more slowly. The amount of oxygen in your body is automatically controlled.

If your heart needs to beat faster or slower, it will do so. Blood flow to the tissues is automatically controlled according to need. These are just a few examples of the many, many control systems in the body. They all have one thing in common: *If a control system is supposed to keep a variable—oxygen, temperature, weight or whatever—at a particular level, **it will keep it at that level!***

We have control systems which help us avoid fatigue, unpleasantness, pain, and discomfort. We have control systems which make us seek protective environments. As our hormonal and reproductive systems mature, we seek mates and reproduce. Thus the very fact that we are alive, survive and reproduce is *almost beyond our control!!* Our control systems are in charge!

Because their mission is to insure our *survival,* our control systems are *extremely powerful.* For that reason it is virtually impossible to override them. Since it is almost impossible to override the control systems of the body, it would seem logical that the best thing to do with them is *use* them to our advantage. That is exactly what you are in the process of doing. You are giving your subconscious, or weight control center, a new setting. It is to control your weight at that new level. You are using the control system to your advantage. Your weight will be automatically controlled at the new level. *You* do the resetting, *it* does the controlling.

It is not uncommon to hear someone say, "If I weighed as much as he/she does, I wouldn't eat another bite until my weight was where it is supposed to be." By making the statement, he is implying that *he* could override one of the body's control systems. Oh yeah? Show me. Look at your watch. Now exhale, relax and don't breathe in any air for 60 seconds. It's difficult? Sure it's difficult! It's just like trying to override any other control system in the body. If you need something (air, water, whatever), your body sends a message that "If you don't get it, you are going to die!" That causes you to have a frantic urge to breathe, drink, whatever. When you do, there is an enormous feeling of relief.

It was difficult to override the control system for respiration, wasn't it? You had trouble overriding a control system for a mere *60 seconds* and you expect someone else to override his for the *rest of his life!* Not likely. He can work to reset it and *use* it, though.

Things to do during Week Eighteen: Continue the process of resetting your appestat. Follow all of the steps. Don't allow your subconscious to perceive you as being any other way except trim. Think of the ancient Greek attitude about eating. Think of their attitude about moderation. Continue to work to eliminate physical and mental stress. Use the visualizations that you have learned. Say "I'm full" whenever you think of the words. Participate in an aerobic activity if you wish.

WEEK NINETEEN

Comments: At this point in your program you need to be aware of some typical statements you are likely to hear from people who know you—particularly people who have known you for a long time. You are changing. It is only natural that others should notice the change. Different individuals will react differently when they do notice.

These are typical of the comments you are likely to hear: "You don't look too good." "Are you sure you're healthy?" "You're not sick, are you?" "You don't look like your old self." "You're losing weight too fast." "You aren't developing that starving disease (anorexia nervosa) are you?" And finally the one you might hear even before you reach the weight you desire, "You don't need to lose any more weight!" It is amazing that anyone would say that to you, but they will. There is a reason.

You may be surprised—even offended—by some of the statements, but consider for a moment what might have prompted individuals to make them. One of the most noticeable features of chronic, debilitating diseases is a progressive decrease in body weight. Cancer is an example. As the cancer cells multiply, they consume more and more of the body's energy. The individual loses weight, looks pale, and becomes weak. The cancerous cells continue to multiply, continue to consume the body's energy until they finally destroy the very host upon which they are dependent. When people who know you see that your weight is decreasing, they may subconsciously think, "illness."

Your weight is decreasing. You don't look pale. You are healthy. You have more energy than you have ever had. You have "energy to burn," but that may not be immediately noticeable to someone who hasn't seen you for a while. If it isn't noticeable, he may be genuinely concerned about your health.

When a person says, "You don't need to lose any more weight," he may be subconsciously saying, "If you do, you'll be thinner than me!"

When a person says, "You don't look like your old self," he may be subconsciously saying, "I don't like change." (You don't look like your old self, you don't want to look like your old self, and you never *will* look like your old self!)

It is important for you to realize that from this point on in your program of body weight adjustment, you are going to hear those statements and other similar statements more and more often. You won't be surprised at them if you are prepared for them. You *will* hear them.

Be patient. Your family and friends will soon discover that you aren't sick. They will discover that you are healthy. They will realize that what you are doing is good for you.

They will soon discover that it is preferable that you look like your "new self" instead of like your "old self."

If it's any consolation to you, after those who know you discover that you're not sick, that you're healthy, that you're energetic and that you're moving your weight to a new level, they will have other comments. They will say, "You look great!" They will ask, "Where did you get all of that energy?" They will ask, "How did you lose all of that weight?"

Tell them.

Things to do during Week Nineteen: Keep your attention focused on your new weight level. Use all of the visualizations. Follow all of the steps. Say the words, "I'm full" to yourself whenever you think about them. Remind yourself that moderation is important, that quality may be preferred to quantity.

WEEK TWENTY

Comments: Beginning with the twentieth week of the program, you are going to "shift gears." You are going to focus on some additional, very positive benefits which will come to you as a result of your continuing in the program.

It is *still important* to keep score just as it was important to keep score as a part of the conditioning process. If you aren't recording your daily score, make a mental note of it at the end of the day. That will constantly remind your appestat of its new duty. This method of constant repetition is necessary to *permanently change* the nerve circuits in the brain.

You are 20 weeks into the program. By now you are "automatically" following the steps necessary to reset your body weight to a new, permanent level! Because you are often subconsciously following the steps, when your body weight does reach the new level, you might have the tendency to think that it "just happened." You might think that it would have gone to a new level even if you had not been on this program. Objectively, of course, you know that your body weight wouldn't have gone to the proper level if you hadn't reset your weight control mechanism.

You have an understanding of how the control systems of the body work. You know that it is folly to try to override them. You have an appreciation of how the appetite control system works. You can see the logic in resetting it and having it work for you instead of trying to work against it by overriding it or fooling it.

You could now very easily teach someone else this method of body weight adjustment. You know that repetition is important in order to permanently change nerve circuits. You have an appreciation of how your own feelings change as you carefully follow the steps to reset your weight control center. You are aware that making certain changes increases life expectancy. You are aware of the benefits to be derived by body weight control. You could also make someone aware of the hazards of some of the "cures" for obesity.

Some new, beneficial information will be brought to your attention for your use (and for you to share with others if, by now, you are helping someone else with the program). Your attention will be focused on the positive effects of being 'slim and trim' and focused on some exciting new possibilities resulting from body weight adjustment.

During this week and the next few weeks, you will be considering information on the *aging* process, life *span* and life *expectancy*. Some of the questions which will be addressed are: What is the aging process? What speeds the aging process? Is there anything that can slow the aging process? Is there anything that can increase the life *expectancy*? Is it possible to increase the life *span*? The answers to some of these questions are going to surprise you!

(Note: You are now doing something which is significantly decreasing the rate at which you are aging and which is significantly increasing your life expectancy: You are losing weight.)

Getting "old" and "aging" aren't necessarily the same. We used to tell people that they had to retire at the age of 65. We'd say, "Okay, you're 65 years old. It's time for you to quit work and start drawing your pension. You're going to die soon." We didn't say it that bluntly, but that, in essence, is the reason we gave for wanting them to retire at that age. Perhaps in years past, that was reason enough, but it no longer is. Today people are living much longer. If we continue to expect individuals to retire at the early age of 65, we need to think of some other reason to give them for wanting them to do so. Our implying "You're going to die soon" is no longer an accurate statement.

(Note: I personally believe that we should eliminate the word "retirement" from our vocabulary, take the word "retirement" out of our dictionary, and remove the concept of "retirement" from our thoughts. I don't mean to imply that we should all stay on the same job as long as we live. After devoting 20 or 30 years to a business or profession, it might well be time for a change—a change, not retirement. You can keep growing those plants that you enjoy; maybe even open a small nursery and share them with your friends. Enroll in art classes—they don't care about your age at college—and paint those pictures you have talked about painting. Dust off that piano, guitar, or other instrument, take some music lessons and write those songs you have talked about writing. If you devote 20 or 30 years to a new endeavor with the same enthusiasm you had when you started your first career, there is no telling where it might lead. Change? Yes, if you wish to. Retire? No. Most truly retired people have a headstone which permanently marks their place of retirement.)

If we persist in telling 65-year-olds to quit work and move to the retirement community, they have every right to say to us "I don't want to quit work. I might consider changing jobs. I might try something new, but I plan to work at least 20 more years. I will probably work for the rest of my life. If I do think about retirement, it's going to be much later. I'm not going to think about it now."

If they feel that way, what are we going to say to them? Perhaps we don't have the answer to that question. If we don't already have an answer, we need to be thinking of one, because we need one now! As individuals continue to make use of the scientific information which is available to them, the majority are going to be living, in good health, well past the age of 90. Is that possible? Is it possible that people are going to keep living longer and longer? It not only is possible, it is now in the process of happening. The life expectancy is increasing with each passing day.

Why is this happening? Probably because of the enormous information explosion which has been occurring in recent years. How does the increased availability of information relate to increased longevity? The information has made new developments possible; it has made it possible for us to completely change our lifestyle, our well-being, our health and our health care delivery. In order to put things more into perspective, let's take a broad look at some of the changes which have taken place in medicine and technology during the past few decades. Let me give you a personal example that will illustrate my point.

My father was born in a rural community soon after the turn of the century. His family home had no electricity, no running water, no central heating, and no refrigeration. Their light came from kerosene lamps, their water from a well, and their heat from wood-burning fireplaces. They had no radios, no television, no supermarkets, and no means of rapid communication. The little-used roads were not paved.

In fact, when my dad was a youngster, he and his family had no better means of transportation than Julius Caesar had had. To be sure, trains and ships existed, but they were not available to them personally as a means of transportation. If he or his family traveled, they either walked, rode a horse or rode in a wagon pulled by horses or mules.

My father and his family tilled the soil with horse-drawn plows. They grew cotton for market and food for themselves and their domesticated animals. They ate potatoes, corn, molasses and seasonal garden vegetables. Farm-raised meat, which was either smoked, salt-cured or, more rarely, canned, was less frequently a part of the daily diet. Occasionally wild game taken from the woods provided a brief respite from the daily fare of "cornbread, beans and greens."

Flour, salt, seasonings, necessary items of clothing, the affordable farm implements and the essential tools were purchased on annual excursions "to town." These trips could be made in "one day." If the family left home at 4 A.M., they could take the cotton to market, purchase the supplies, and be back home by 10 o'clock that night. Not bad, considering that they had to travel a distance of nearly 20 miles just to get to town.

There is no doubt that technology fared poorly a few decades ago; medicine probably fared worse.

The life expectancy of a person born soon after the turn of the century was short compared to present-day standards and very short when one considers that the human life span is now probably about 110 years. Only 41 percent of the people born in 1900 could expect to reach the age of 65. During those times people died of appendicitis, pneumonia, typhoid fever, scarlet fever, smallpox and other infectious diseases. Cardiovascular diseases and cancer were rampant then, as they are now.

The delivery of health care was almost nonexistent. If one summoned a physician, about all the physician had to offer was his presence, charm and personality. The use of analgesics and anesthetics was antiquated. Antibiotics were nonexistent. Those deficiencies often made surgery more hazardous to the patient than the disease with which the patient was afflicted.

My father was bitten on the foot by a snake when he was a young boy. Someone, probably one of the other boys, was sent to bring the doctor. A day or so later, the doctor—a circuit-riding physician—arrived, examined the swollen extremity and decided on a course of treatment. He placed a ball of cotton on the wound, put a few drops of liquid—probably alcohol—on the cotton and set it afire in order to "draw out" the poison. The ensuing pain did serve to divert my father's attention from his encounter with the reptile, but the treatment accomplished little else. He managed to recover both from his unfortunate accident and from the ineffective healing rites which were inflicted upon him. The physician received profuse thanks from the family, some small gratuity—probably a laying hen—and was on his way to attend the next crisis. My father survived those early years on the farm. As of this writing, he is an alert 83-year old.

Such was the state of technology and the practice of medicine a few short years ago. Today, one little freckle-faced kid on a big International Harvester tractor pulling a gang of plows can turn over more dirt after he comes home from school than 100 laborers with hoes could turn over in a day's time back then. Air travel makes it possible to have breakfast in Atlanta and lunch in San Francisco. Instant communication to almost any point on the planet is possible. Satellites circle the earth. Others probe our solar system and beyond. Live television coverage from the most remote corners of the world is commonplace. A multitude of devices have been developed to wash, cook, clean, heat, cool, dry, humidify, deodorize, sanitize, mobilize and entertain. Creature comforts abound. Miraculous computers chew up problems and spit out solutions. Much of our energy today is directed at obtaining additional luxuries, not at mere survival. Our increase in productivity is mind-boggling. Technology has truly come alive during recent years. We have seen only the beginning. Conditions are such, at this point in time, that we can lead longer, more productive lives.

Medicine, too, has made a transition. There has been a revolution in medicine and in the delivery of medical care. Today, thanks to a flurry of activity in medical research laboratories during the past 40 years, the physician can deliver the cure for many diseases and the prevention and treatment of many others. Some diseases which wreaked havoc on many lives just a few short years ago, are almost nonexistent today. The life expectancy is now well past 70 years and is headed toward 80. It will continue to go higher. Soon after the turn of the century, the life expectancy will likely exceed 90 years.

In recent times the development of antibiotics has made it possible to combat infectious diseases. The development of vaccines has led to the effective treatment of other diseases, and to the virtual elimination of diseases—such as polio and smallpox—which were once both crippling and deadly.

New drugs continually appear on the market. Drugs for treating high blood pressure; drugs for thinning the blood to prevent the formation of damaging blood clots; promising drugs which may be able to alter the blood fat level; drugs for treating pain, infection, inflammatory process, and a multitude of other types of medication are now a part of the physician's ammunition for treating diseases.

Artificial heart valves, synthetic artery grafts, machines for taking over the circulation of blood during open-heart surgery, and artificial kidney machines have all been developed during the past few years. Refined surgical procedures are continually being developed. Open-heart surgery is commonplace. New eye, brain, and bone surgical techniques are available, as are new techniques in all of the surgical disciplines.

In addition, new diagnostic equipment abounds. Scanning of the body with computerized axial tomography (CAT-scan) is a widely used new technique. It allows a gathering of anatomical information—a look at the cross-section of the body—presented as an image generated by a computer. The computer receives information from a number of x-ray transmissions, synthesizes the information, and presents it on a screen as a cross-section of the body. The CAT-scan makes it possible to actually identify small (and large) normal and abnormal anatomical structures inside the body without surgically invading the body.

Positron emission tomography (PET) makes possible the imaging of metabolic and physiological functions in the body. The fact that we can "visualize" chemical reactions in the body staggers the imagination. The image is formed by a computerized synthesis of data transmitted by positron-emitting substances that have been incorporated into natural biochemicals and given to the patient. Computer analysis of the data shows up as different colors (or the absence of colors). The different colors, or the absence of colors, represent the rate of metabolism (energy usage) in specific tissues. The presence or absence of disease can be determined by examining the different colors.

The death rate from heart disease in the United States has dropped 40 percent in the last 20 years. (According to the American Heart Association, lifestyle changes alone can cut the *current* death rate in half!) Better methods of diagnosis and treatment are partially responsible for the 40 percent decrease in deaths from heart disease, but changes in lifestyle, such as eating diets lower in fats, controlling blood pressure, smoking less, and getting more exercise, have all interacted to dramatically reduce the death rates. The death rate from heart disease in the United States will continue to drop as our lifestyles continue to change.

None of these amazing developments in the field of medicine "just happened." They came as a result of a calculated all-out assault on a group of diseases which cause humans to die before they have lived out their life span. Activities in the medical research laboratories, although slowed in recent years by budgetary restrictions, are continuing at a very rapid pace.

All of the changes in medicine and technology noted above have taken place in a very short period of time. They occurred in just the past few decades. That's phenomenal, considering that humans have been on this planet for thousands of years. Additional, more dramatic breakthroughs are on the horizon. New developments are likely to occur more rapidly in the future than they have in the past. Will we grow to accept the remarkable as commonplace? Probably.

Getting "old" is a state of mind. People are getting "old" later in life than they used to. Decide for yourself on an advanced age that you consider "old." Decide that you will get "old" only after you reach that age. If you don't consciously select a particular age that you consider "old," your subconscious will select one for you. That could work to your disadvantage. Here's why. In times past, the age of 50 was considered "old." At that age one was supposed to begin to "take it easy" so as not to "overdo it." People were admonished not to "overwork the heart." It was assumed that joints would stiffen, muscles would weaken, and the capacity for productive endeavors would rapidly decline. It became a self-fulfilling prophecy. When people took it easy, those things happened. When limbs were not moved, joints stiffened; when muscles were not contracted, they became weaker; and when energy was not expended, the capacity for productivity decreased. Sure enough, by the time people reached the age of 50, they were old! They weren't surprised. They thought they were *supposed* to be old by then.

More recently it has become fashionable to be "old" at a later age. Bureaucratic benevolence has made it possible for people to retire at the age of 65—or at 62 if one chooses to take "early retirement." This somewhat arbitrary assignment of "old age" and "senior citizen" status to millions of people was done by congressmen who often continue to work after they are well into their 80s. Surprisingly, we complied with their decision! We stopped getting old at 50 and began getting old at 65! Instead of having stiffened joints, weaker muscles and reduced capacity for productivity at the age of 50, we postponed those conditions until we were 65. How remarkable! Isn't it time some farsighted individuals decided that changes should be postponed even longer—that they should take place even later in life than at the age of 65? How about postponing getting old until the age of 85, or 95 or 105? Why not? It has been postponed once; it can be postponed again.

For the moment, resolve that when you do focus on an age when you are going to "get old," your attention will be on the goal and not on "what will happen if" you get old before you reach it. "What will happen if" has kept many people from reaching goals. Here is an old story about deciding whether to focus on a goal or on the consequences of not achieving it. You may remember the story; it goes like this:

Suppose I find a nice strong oak board that is about 20 feet long, two feet wide and four inches thick. I place the board on the lawn in front of the house and place some money— enough for you to have an evening out—on one end of it. I then offer to give you the money if you walk the length of the board, without stepping off, and pick the money up. No problem! The board is two feet wide. You could probably walk it with your eyes closed. Besides, it would be no big deal if you did happen to get distracted and step off. So without hesitation you walk it and pick up the money. You didn't come close to stepping off. You didn't even think about stepping off. You were thinking about picking up the money. You were focusing on your goal . . . But now let's change things. Let's put one end of that same board on top of a ten-story building and the other end across the alley to the top of another ten-story building. I put the same amount of money at the end of the board and offer it to you if you walk the length of the board again. Would you do it? Why not? It's just as wide as before. You have to walk the same distance to get the money. What's the difference? The difference is that now with the board on top of the buildings, you can't concentrate on the goal for concentrating on the "What if?"

When you make up your mind to "get old" at a later age—much later than 65—resolve to think only about that. You don't want the "what if" to get in the way.

Aging. Aging produces changes in the structure and function of the body. All animals, humans included, change continually from birth to death. After they are born, a variable period of time is required for them to mature. Following maturation, they continue to change until the end of their lives. Aging occurs faster in some animal species than it does in other species. It progresses faster in some humans than it does in other humans. (See Figure 7.)

Turtles—the Galapagos tortoise, for example—may live for more than 200 years. The laboratory rat lives approximately two to three years. The life span of humans is somewhere between the two. It is not uncommon for humans to live for 100 or more years. It is a fact that the aging process does occur faster in some animal species than it does in others.

Why do turtles live for 200 years, humans for 100 years and laboratory rats for three years? The simple answer is that the mechanism which governs the aging process operates at different speeds in each of the three different species. This fact provides a useful clue.

Some signs of aging in the human are obvious. There is wrinkling of the skin, loss of muscle mass, decrease in muscle strength, loss or graying of hair, increase in fat deposits, and decrease in endurance. These are *programmed* changes. Humans don't "wear out" simply due to the passage of time. These changes don't occur simply because a person "gets older." If the human "aging clock" is not functioning properly, all of these changes can occur *while an individual is still very young*.

Some of the signs of aging are not so obvious as those mentioned above. Whether the signs are obvious or not, the ultimate effects of aging are related to (1) a decrease in the total number of cells in the body and (2) a progressive decrease in the function of the cells which remain. When viewed in this light, it doesn't seem so far-fetched to believe that something can be done about the aging process. The specifics of what that "something" is will be spelled out in coming weeks.

By reducing your body weight, you are slowing the progressive decrease in the function of the cells and organs of your body.

Next week some other effects of aging will be considered. These effects include changes in the cardiovascular, digestive, hormonal, and other systems, changes which are not as obvious as the wrinkling of the skin or the accumulation of fat deposits. If the "aging clock" is not functioning properly, these systems can also age extremely rapidly while an individual is still very young.

Things to do during Week Twenty: (1) Say to yourself, "I am slim and trim" as often as appropriate. (2) Visualize yourself as trim. (3) Continue to engage in some type of physical activity. (4) Think of the attitude that the ancient Greeks had about eating. (5) Say to yourself, "I'm full" whenever it is appropriate. (6) Realize that you are changing your self-image.

Chapter 8

Does Weight Reduction Prolong Youth?
(Weeks 21–26)

WEEK TWENTY-ONE

Comments: Since a decrease in the total number of cells in the body and a decrease in the function of the cells which remain are the characteristics of the aging process, it follows that all of the systems in the body are affected by aging. As mentioned earlier, some of the effects of aging are easily noticeable. Others aren't.

Changes which occur with age in the different systems of the body are given below. Next week some ways to inhibit those changes will be discussed.

Let's consider the skeletal system first. Calcium is lost from the bones with age. The calcium loss begins earlier in women than in men. It begins sometime around the age of 40 in women and after the age of 60 in men. As aging progresses, the bones are less capable of producing protein, one of bones' structural components. Consequently the bones become more brittle and more susceptible to fracture.

The muscular system is also affected by aging. Muscle cells are continually lost as individuals get older, and there is a decrease in the maximum strength of muscle contraction. These changes usually begin after the age of 30 in both men and women and continue for the remainder of life. The lost muscle tissue is normally replaced by fat. There is a decrease in the speed of muscle reflexes which is due to the aging of both the muscular and nervous systems.

As individuals get older, the heart also tends to become weaker. It can't pump as much blood as it previously could.

Hardening of the arteries progresses with age. If a major artery which supplies blood to the heart muscle becomes "clogged," a heart attack will result. If arteries supplying blood to the brain become "clogged," a person will have a small or large stroke, depending on the size of the vessels which are clogged. The brain cells supplied by the vessels will die. The blood pressure tends to rise with age so that a person who had a normal blood pressure earlier in life might become hypertensive later in life.

The primary effect of aging on the nervous system is the loss of nerve cells. The result is a decrease in the ability to send impulses to and from the brain and a decrease in ability to send them from place to place within the brain. The speed at which the nerve impulses travel slows with age. This, coupled with a progressive decrease in muscle strength, results in a slowing of the reflexes of the body. The effects of aging on the nerve cells also alter the sensations of sight, smell, taste, touch and hearing.

Another system affected by aging is the endocrine system. The endocrine system produces hormones. A variety of changes occurs in this system as individuals get older. Basically, aging results in a reduction in the amount of the various hormones which are produced. This doesn't cause major problems unless the hormonal production is severely curtailed. (Example: If, as an individual gets older, the body doesn't produce enough insulin, diabetes develops.) Many investigators believe that further study of the endocrine system will reveal the secret to the aging process.

As an individual gets older, the respiratory system changes in several ways. The airways and the air sacs in the lung become less elastic. This means that they can't expand and contract as much when a person breathes in and out. The walls of the chest become more rigid with age. As a result of both of these changes, there is a decrease in the amount of air that the lungs can hold. If you breathe in as much air as you can, then blow out as much air as you can, that volume of air is called the vital capacity. The vital capacity may decrease by as much as 35 to 40 percent by the time a person reaches the age of 70.

With advancing age, the digestive system produces fewer secretions and enzymes necessary for the digestive process. The muscles in the wall of the digestive tract lose some of their strength. This results in reduced muscular movement to churn and propel the contents through the digestive tract. Both digestion and absorption become less efficient as individuals get older.

Aging affects the filtering ability of the kidneys. Each person normally has two kidneys, and each kidney has approximately one million filtering units (nephrons). Survival is possible with only one-third of that number of nephrons. By the time an individual has reached the age of 70, the number of nephrons may be reduced to one-half of their original number. That is a sufficient number to do the job (with plenty to spare) as long as major kidney diseases are avoided.

Both the male and female reproductive systems change with age. In both sexes, fertility decreases with age. There is a decrease in the production of the "female hormones" (progesterone and estrogens). In the male there is reduced production of the "male hormone" (testosterone). The number of sperm cells is reduced although abundant sperm cells may be found even in old age.

As the above information indicates, changes occur in all of the major systems of the body as individuals age. Are all of the changes "inevitable?" No, they're not. Some of the changes that occur have been identified. That is important, since it is necessary to identify a problem before a solution can be sought. It is necessary to identify the things that do happen before measures can be sought which might inhibit them. For years scientists have been doing both.

It is possible to inhibit some of the changes brought on by the aging process. As a matter of fact, you are already inhibiting the aging process by adjusting your body weight to a lower level. You are enhancing the ability of many of the systems in your body to perform longer and more efficiently. How are you doing that? More details will be given in coming weeks along with information on other ways to inhibit some of the effects of aging.

Things to do during Week Twenty-One: This week you will be given an additional phrase to use *while you are eating*. (Note: If you have read ahead in this book and haven't progressed to WEEK TWENTY-ONE, don't start using the phrase early. Wait until you are in WEEK TWENTY-ONE to use it.)

Do you remember when you were young and your mother plopped down a big helping of something on your plate and said, "Now eat it all. It's good for you"? You probably said—if not aloud to your mother then at least to yourself—"Do I *have* to eat it *all*?" Almost everyone can remember a similar experience. The statement that you made to your mother (or to yourself) then can become a useful one now. Here's how:

Continue to follow all of the steps in your resetting program including saying to yourself, "I'm full." *In addition,* while you are eating, when you do begin to feel full, look at the remaining food on your plate and say to yourself, "Do I have to eat it *all*?" The answer, of course, is "No you *don't* have to eat it all!" You can do as you wish. You can eat it or not eat it. Ask yourself the question, "Do I have to eat it all?" several times. Then do as you choose.

If you included activity as a part of your program, be sure to mention it in your comments each day. If you walked, log it. If you swam, rode a bike or participated in any other activity, log it. That will allow you to periodically review and assess your progress.

WEEK TWENTY-TWO

Comments: As the different systems of the body age, the body becomes more vulnerable to disease. The body also becomes susceptible to internal and external stress. Thus it is desirable for health as well as for cosmetic reasons to inhibit all of the aging processes as much as possible.

Last week changes which occur with age in the different systems of the body were described. Beginning this week, methods of inhibiting those changes will be discussed. Since one of the most noticeable effects of aging is the effect it has on the skin, that effect will be considered first.

The skin and the associated structures of the skin—hair, nails and glands—are constantly aging, as are all of the other systems of the body. The aging effect doesn't become particularly noticeable until the late 40s. Why does the skin age? There are white fibers of connective tissue (called collagen) in the skin which are made of protein. There are also elastic fibers of connective tissue in the skin; with age these fibers fray and break. As a result the skin wrinkles. There are cells in the skin called fibroblasts. The fibroblasts produce both collagen and elastic fibers, but their numbers decrease with age. The oil glands of the skin atrophy and atypical skin pigmentation may occur.

Prolonged exposure to ultraviolet rays from the sun will speed the aging process. Also, molecules known as "free radicals" can weaken protein. Free radicals are particular types of oxygen molecules with free electrons on them. As the normal metabolic processes of the body take place, these free radicals flail about inside and outside the cells of the body, destroying them and thus aging us. Radiation and toxic agents produce free radicals. On the other hand—and this is very important as regards prevention—certain substances inhibit the formation of free radicals. Vitamin E, which is found in vegetable oils and whole grain cereals; vitamin C, which is found in fresh fruits and vegetables; and the element selenium, which is found in meats, seafood and grains, all inhibit the formation of free radicals.

Some sagging of the skin with age may be the result of a loss of muscle tone and not due to the aging process at all. Restoring muscle tone will eliminate that.

There are many oils, creams, lotions and "formulas" which claim to help you retain the youthful appearance of the skin. By early 1987, cosmetic companies were making such exaggerated claims for their products that the FDA warned a multitude of them—including many of the "name" companies—to stop making claims which had no scientific basis. They should have stopped making the claims. The fact is, the skin over most of the body is five layers thick. The aging process takes place *beneath* those layers, and it is unlikely that lotions and oils reach that deep. However, they might moisturize the surface of the skin and make you feel good. The three things that *really inhibit the aging of the skin* are: avoiding long exposure to radiation; eating foods which are conducive to good skin health; and maintaining muscle tone.

The second system which will be examined during WEEK TWENTY-TWO is the skeletal system.

As mentioned earlier, calcium is lost from the bones beginning after age 40 in women and after age 60 in men. Many physicians prescribe calcium supplementation in the form of two calcium-containing antiacid tablets daily when additional calcium is needed. That is an inexpensive way to obtain additional calcium. Bone meal is commonly used as a calcium supplement, although it may not be the best source. In a 1986 report to the American Society of Pharmacology and Experimental Therapeutics, Boulos and Smolinski showed that traces of lead were found in bone meal tablets which were purchased from a health food store over a six-month period. Calcium-containing foods are the best source of calcium.

Inactivity speeds the demineralization process of the skeletal system as a result of the lack of stress it imparts to the bones. (The term "stress" is used here to indicate pressure or tension on the bones, in contrast to "stress" which may be put on the bones by various disease processes.) The blood level of calcium increases soon after cessation of activity, indicating that the demineralization process quickly follows inactivity. This can occur in healthy individuals. It happens to astronauts if they don't exercise when they are exposed to weightlessness. The effects of the aging process on the bones can be inhibited by (1) calcium supplementation when needed and (2) actively stressing the bones by some type of daily exercise. Bones are stressed as a result of weight-bearing by standing upright and by muscle contraction during physical activity.

Methods of inhibiting the effects of aging on the muscular system will be discussed next week.

Things to do during Week Twenty-Two: Last week you were given an additional phrase to use. While you are eating, when you begin to feel full, look at the remaining food on your plate and ask yourself the question, "Do I *have* to eat it all?" Ask yourself the question several times, then do as you choose.

Continue to apply the other steps. Remember, it is *repetition* that permanently changes the nerve circuits. Apply the other steps, record your score and record your comments when appropriate.

By recording your comments, you can look back and recall your feelings at a particular time in the program. This may be especially useful if you are helping someone else with the program. If you are helping someone else with the program, remind them to use the visualization regarding moderation in living and eating.

WEEK TWENTY-THREE

Comments: Have you ever seen a youngster who had to wear a cast because of a broken bone? When the cast was removed after a period of time, the muscles underneath were smaller and weaker than similar muscles on the other side of the body. This type of decrease in muscle size is known as disuse atrophy. That is, the muscle became smaller and weaker because of a lack of use. Exercise will restore such muscles to their normal size and strength. Disuse atrophy is also sometimes seen in people who are getting older. It might be mistaken for atrophy due to aging, when in reality the muscles have gotten smaller and weaker simply because they have been used less. Muscle cells are continually lost as individuals get older. The maximum strength of contraction also decreases. But much of what we see in the way of decrease in muscle size and strength with age is the result of what we see in a child with a cast—disuse atrophy.

If muscles are stretched daily, if tension is put on them daily, if they receive the proper nutrition, then the effects which we ordinarily associate with aging will be inhibited. It is not necessary to work out in a gymnasium or fitness center daily. The majority of individuals do not have access to such facilities nor the time to use them if they had access to them. Tension can be put on muscles by walking, by climbing a few steps, or by lifting an object, such as a large book, several times a day. Have you ever seen animals—cats or dogs—stretch after they wake up from a nap? They are stretching and putting tension on their muscles and giving their joints the full range of motion. They are getting ready for action.

Tension can be put on muscle groups in any number of ways. Here is an example of how you can take a few seconds of time to put tension on some muscle groups. Hold your left hand out in front of you, palm side up. Grasp it, palm to palm, with your right hand. Now bring your clasped hands to your chest and back to waist level several times as you offer resistance to the movement. Do this a few times, then turn your right palm up and do the same thing. You can think of similar ways to offer resistance to other muscle groups in your body. Include activity which can be incorporated into your daily routine. For example, to tighten your abdominal muscles, sit on the floor with your toes under a couch or heavy chair. Now lie on your back with your arms folded across your chest. Contract your abdominal muscles as if you were going to sit up—it is not necessary to sit all the way up in order to contract the muscles. Walking is an exercise for the legs, trunk, and respiratory muscles.

The above are just some examples of ways to put tension on muscle groups. These and other repetitious exercises which offer resistance to the different muscle groups of the body will inhibit the effects which are often thought to be due to aging.

Repetitious joint movements can help maintain joint flexibility and at the same time can stretch the different muscle groups. Giving the full range of motion—or as near thereto as possible—to the various joints of the body each day requires little time or effort. It can be easily incorporated into one's daily activities. Believing that joint motion just naturally decreases with age becomes a self-fulfilling prophecy if the joints are allowed to stiffen because of infrequent movement.

Simple exercises can provide a full range of motion to the joints of the body. Here are some: Extending the arms at the sides and making small circles which progressively become larger circles increases the flexibility of the shoulder. Slowly rolling the head from side to side loosens the joints of the neck. Leaning from side to side moves the spine and stretches the muscles of the side of the body. Rotating the hand and the foot loosens the wrist and ankle joints. Sitting in a chair and extending the legs back and forth loosens the muscles of the thigh and gives a good range of motion to the knee joint. The elbow joints can be loosened by extending the arms to the side and bringing the hands up to touch the shoulders. Hip joint flexiblity can be increased by holding to the back of a chair and extending the leg first forward, then backward. Standing on the tiptoes exercises the muscles of the lower leg and works the ankles. Sitting in a chair and leaning forward stretches the lower back muscles.

These motions will stretch muscles and maintain joint flexiblity. They are things that you can do *every day* for as long as you live. You don't have to go to a gym to do them; they can be incorporated into your daily routine. The motions are simple to do. Repetitious exercises which help maintain joint flexibility will inhibit changes in joints which are often thought to be due to aging.

Eating the proper food is also important in inhibiting the aging of muscles. A certain amount of carbohydrate in the diet is required to provide the body with a simple sugar (glucose). Glucose is the body's basic energy source. If diets are very high in protein and very low in carbohydrate, the body attempts to obtain the glucose from stored fat. This causes fatty acids in the body to be incompletely broken down. If the body is not getting enough carbohydrate in the diet and fatty acids are incompletely broken down, the body must obtain glucose from other sources. Unfortunately the other sources are the muscles and the major body organs such as the heart. This process can result in a decrease in muscle size which may be mistaken for shrinkage due to aging. In other words, *the muscles need a balanced diet*. Clarification of the term "balanced diet" will be a part of next week's comments.

In summary, the effects of aging on the muscular system can be inhibited by (1) the daily *application* of *tension* to the different *muscle groups* in the form of activity which you make a part of your daily routine and (2) a diet which insures an adequate intake of carbohydrates so that the body's basic energy source, glucose, will be available for use. With proper diet, the body will not be required to draw upon the muscles and other organs for the needed glucose.

Things to do during Week Twenty-Three: Try stretching your muscles and putting tension on different muscle groups *as you go about your daily routine*. Give a full range of motion to your joints.

This is an appropriate time in your body weight adjustment program to reaffirm your commitment to following the steps necessary to *reset* your subconscious, or weight control center. As you acquire new information about the body and its function, continue to follow the steps in the program. Look at your reflection and tell yourself that you are slim and trim. Visualize yourself as being trim. *Know* in your mind that you are trim. While you are eating, say the words "I'm full" to yourself to let your subconscious or weight control center know that it is okay for you not to feel hungry even though you are now much smaller than you once were.

Remember, as you follow these steps, you are changing your body weight to a new level and inhibiting the aging process.

WEEK TWENTY-FOUR

Comments: The digestive system changes with age. The changes include a decrease in the amount of the secretions necessary for digestion and a decrease in the muscular movement (motility). These two changes can lead to some other problems with the digestive system; problems such as maldigestion, malabsorption, constipation, and gastritis.

Three items head the list of things which may speed the aging process of the digestive system: (1) toxic substances, (2) improper diets, and (3) improper eating habits. It follows then that several things can be done to *inhibit* the aging process of the digestive system. Let us take in order the three items mentioned above: First, individuals should, as much as possible, avoid the ingestion of toxic substances. What are some examples of toxic substances? Trihalomethane from improperly purified water; chlorinated hydrocarbons from industral pollution; lead from old lead water pipes; and heavy metals such as cadmium and mercury from contaminated foods are all examples of toxic substances. Alcohol, when consumed in excess, is a toxic substance. In short, anything that is not nutritious, required food and drink should be considered potentially toxic. That doesn't necessarily mean that everything that you eat should be "natural." Remember, lead, arsenic and poison ivy are "natural." Just because something is natural doesn't automatically make it good for you.

Eating a proper diet is also important if the effect of aging on the digestive system is to be inhibited. Basically there are four food groups: (1) fruits and vegetables; (2) grains and cereals; (3) meats; (4) dairy products. Selection of items from each of the four groups will give one a "balance" to his daily intake of food. An adequate vitamin intake can be assured by having at least one serving of a dark green or a dark yellow vegetable plus fresh fruit, daily if possible, but at least every other day. Fruits, which some individuals use as desserts, should be fresh if possible and the vegetables should be eaten raw when appropriate. Meat which is broiled or steamed is better for you than fried meats. Visible fat should be trimmed from meat before it is cooked. If you choose to include red meats such as pork and beef in your diet, you probably won't want to have them more than three times a week. Even then it will be better if you choose the very leanest cuts. The fourth food group, dairy products, should be low-fat items such as skim milk and low-fat cheese. This group of foods provides the required calcium and riboflavin in your diet. Riboflavin is one of the heat stable factors of the vitamin B complex. Deficiencies may cause inflammation of the mucous membranes which line the mouth, and may also cause some skin problems.

While it is easy to say that selection of items from each of the four food groups will give one a "balance" to the daily intake of food, more specific information about the amount to select from each group is necessary if one is to eat a balanced diet. The body needs proteins, carbohydrates and fats. You should get approximately 15 percent of your daily calories from proteins, 60 percent from carbohydrates and the remaining 25 percent from fats. The average person in the U.S. gets more than 40 percent of his daily calories from fats. That percentage is far too high. (More about fats later.)

It isn't that difficult to obtain 15 percent of the daily intake of calories from proteins. Proteins are found in meat, fish, dairy products, and legumes such as peas and beans. Most animal-derived proteins contain all of the essential amino acids, while some of the vegetable-derived ones do not. (If you are a vegetarian and obtaining all of your proteins from vegetable sources, select a variety of protein-containing foods so that you will get all of the essential amino acids.)

A 150-pound adult requires approximately 50 to 60 grams (about two ounces) of protein daily. Perhaps that doesn't sound like very much—and it may seem unimportant—but protein is essential for growth, repair and maintenance of the body. Even so, more is not always better. Excess protein intake may contribute to health problems such as obesity, particularly if the excess proteins are obtained from animal-derived foods. Those foods are a good source of protein but they also contain a lot of fat.

Carbohydrates are found in foods such as breads, potatoes, rice, beans, and pasta. They should provide most of your daily calories, and they serve as a quick energy source. Insufficient intake will lead to malaise, malnutrition, and the use of some of the body's vital proteins for energy.

The average person obtains too many of his daily calories from fats, but some fat in the diet is necessary. Fat is stored in the body and converted to energy if needed. The cells of the body need some fat in order to function normally. The optimum amount of fat in the diet is an amount which will provide 20 to 30 percent of the total calories. Excess fat in the diet is linked to obesity, heart disease, and cancer. There are different kinds of fats. Animal-derived foods contain saturated fats while the fat found in vegetables is polyunsaturated. (The latter is preferred.) Severe restriction of fat intake will lead to malnutrition, although this is a rare type of malnutrition in the U.S.

The proper selection of food from the four food groups will provide needed fiber in the diet. The recommended minimum daily intake of fiber for an adult is 40 grams. Fiber aids in the passage of materials through the digestive tract. It also binds fat which is in the digestive tract. Low levels of fiber in the diet are associated with disorders such as colon cancer and diverticulosis. Wheat, vegetables, fruits, and grains contain fiber. (A serving of bran cereal contains 10–12 grams of fiber and a large apple contains 5 grams.)

One would not wish to oversimplify what is meant by a "balanced" diet. Yet sometimes something is needed that is not cumbersome to remember. Perhaps the following few sentences will serve that purpose.

[Remember to concentrate on getting enough fresh fruits and vegetables, carbohydrates, fiber, and calcium. Eat enough protein to provide the essential amino acids and 15 percent of your daily calories. Some fat in the diet is necessary, but limit it to 15 to 30 percent of your daily calories.]

What are the vegetables, fruits, carbohydrates, proteins, fats and fiber-containing foods that one might eat in order to achieve and maintain good health? Some *examples* are given below:

1. The nonstarchy vegetables are the foods which have the fewest calories and are high in vitamins and minerals. They also contain fiber and calcium. The nonstarchy vegetables include: broccoli, cabbage, carrots, eggplant, greens, green beans, lettuce, okra, squash, tomatoes, and zucchini. (At least one serving per day.)

2. Fruits which provide fiber and which provide vitamin C when eaten raw include: apples, bananas, blackberries, cantaloupe, grapefruit, grapes, oranges, nectarines, peaches, pears, pineapple, raisins, and strawberries. (One or two servings per day.)

3. Carbohydrates may be obtained from several foods, including: bread, blackeyed peas, corn, English peas, lima beans, potatoes, rice, rolls, and spaghetti. (These are examples of foods which contain carbohydrates; there are many others. Sixty percent of your daily calories should come from carbohydrates. If you consume 1800 calories each day, carbohydrates should provide 1080 of them.)

4. Protein sources include: cheese (low-fat is better for you), chicken, fish, tuna, and turkey. Beef, lamb, pork, and veal contain protein, but these foods should be eaten in limited quantities because of the fat content. You may also obtain protein from grains, beans, peas, and other legumes. (The average adult requires approximately 2 ounces of protein daily.)

5. Fat is found in salad dressings, oils, mayonnaise, margarine, nuts, and meats. (Since the average person in the U.S. gets 40 percent of his calories from fats, most of us probably need to *reduce* our fat intake rather than worrying about whether or not we are getting 25 percent of our calories from fat.)

6. Sources of fiber, in addition to the fruits and vegetables listed above, include bran muffins, bran buds, corn flakes,

shredded wheat, and other wheat cereals.

Q. Is it necessary that I follow a diet such as this in order to lose weight?

A. No, it is not necessary. The current discussion is concerned with ways to inhibit the effects of aging on the digestive system (and on the other systems of the body). The diet outlined above is helpful in that respect. It will also assist one in achieving and maintaining good health. (Remember, you lose weight by changing your appestat, not by dieting.)

The third item mentioned which adversely affects the digestive system is improper eating habits. What constitutes *proper* eating habits? If some attention is given to regularity and tranquility, you are on a safe course. If you can eat at approximately the same time each day in a relaxed atmosphere, you will be doing your digestive system a favor.

You may find the following sequence of events interesting: As individuals lose weight, they become more physically active. When they become more physically active, they tend to eat a balanced diet. They increase their intake of nutritious foods. They often find that they, as active thin people, are actually eating *more* than they were when they were overweight and inactive! They keep their digestive system highly activated. By doing so they probably prolong its vigor and inhibit the effect aging has on it.

You lose weight by changing your appestat and not by dieting, but you can help your appestat by eating a balanced diet. Since the amount of food that you eat is determined by whether your appestat sends out the message "I'm full" or whether it sends out the message "I'm hungry," it is desirable that your appestat be easily satisfied when you have eaten the proper number of calories.

A balanced diet will help in that regard because the appestat responds both to the number of calories consumed and to the type of food that one eats in order to obtain the calories. We probably subconsciously know this, but sometimes we have a tendency to starve ourselves, believing that we will be thin as a result of having done so. Let's examine the interaction of the appestat and a balanced diet a bit further.

If a person who weighs 130 pounds and is physically active requires 2,000 calories a day, he might obtain the calories in any number of ways. To use a far-fetched example, he could, if his digestive system didn't protest too strongly, get all 2,000 calories by eating 10 ounces of pure butter once a day. Or he could get his 2,000 calories by eating 14 pounds of broccoli a day. The appestat would not be permanently satisfied in either case. These are extreme examples, of course, but the *opposite* of these extremes is that a *balanced* diet, eaten at regular intervals during one's waking hours, will more easily satisfy the appestat.

Since a balanced diet will more easily satisfy the appestat, the incredible, inescapable conclusion to be drawn from that fact is this: *Stop dieting, eat a balanced diet, and lose weight!* Believe it or not, that is exactly what has happened to a number of people. When they started eating a balanced diet—a diet containing 60–70 percent carbohydrates, 15–20 percent protein, and 15–20 percent fat—and began eating regular meals, they became more "tuned in" to their appestat. The appestat was better able to communicate its messages; better able to respond to the needs of the body; and better able to adjust the body weight to the proper level.

If you were to put on earphones and listen to a recording that said, "I'm full, I'm full" 24 hours a day, day after day, you would probably get to the point that you wouldn't eat anything at all. Your appestat would become completely fatigued after it sent out the message "I'm hungry" for a long period of time and failed to get a response. Once it quit sending out the message, you would quit being hungry. That is an undesirable situation because of the potentially disastrous results. The program outlined in this book allows you to send the message, "I'm full" to your appestat, and allows you to send other messages and visualization to your appestat at a frequency sufficient to bring the setting of your appestat in line with your body's needs. By resetting your appestat, you will continue to seek food when your body needs it, and you will not seek food when it isn't necessary that you eat.

When one considers all that has been learned about the appestat, one comes to the conclusion that the PRIMARY LAW for attaining and maintaining the proper body weight is: *Reset the Appestat.* That can be done by sending messages and visualization to the appestat. Although that is all that is required, there are some *assist* procedures which facilitate the process of resetting the appestat. They are: (1) stop dieting; (2) eat a balanced diet; (3) engage in a daily program of physical activity (such as walking).

To prevent premature aging of the digestive system: (1) avoid ingesting toxic substances; (2) eat a balanced diet from the four food groups; and (3) form proper eating habits.

Endocrine System. The endocrine system produces hormones. Basically, aging results in a reduction in the amount of the various hormones which are produced. Ordinarily this doesn't cause problems. Most of the disorders of the endocrine system and most of the difficulties which individuals encounter are a result of disease and not advancing age. Prolonged stress adversely affects the endocrine system. You are in the process of *significantly* reducing the stress on your endocrine system by adjusting your body weight to a new level. This may be *the single most important thing* you could do for your endocrine system now to inhibit the aging process. You are also reducing the stress on your endocrine system if you have been practicing getting rid of the mental stressors such as worry and guilt (stressors which don't change things anyway).

Things to do during Week Twenty-Four: Continue to follow all of the steps in your resetting process including saying to yourself "I'm full" whenever you think about it and especially while you are eating. In addition, while you are eating, when you do begin to feel full, look at the remaining food on your plate and say to yourself, "Do I *have* to eat it *all*?" Use all of the visualizations which are available to you. Keep the image of yourself as a trim person firmly fixed in your mind.

Record your points each day. The repetition is necessary to permanently change the nerve circuits. Record your thoughts under "comments" *when appropriate*. In other words, don't feel compelled to write something every day. Jot down your thoughts when they occur to you so you can refer back to them if you wish or so you can refer to them if you are helping someone with this program. Log your activity.

WEEK TWENTY-FIVE

Comments: Let us now take a look at some ways to inhibit the aging of the cardiovascular system. Some effective scientifically verified methods for prolonging the health of the cardiovascular system have been developed. Since *48 percent* of Americans die of heart and blood vessel diseases, a lot of time has been devoted to the study of this system. Much has been learned about it. If you are going to give priority to inhibiting the aging of any particular system of the body, the cardiovascular system should be at or near the top of the list of the ones being considered. It can be injured just as any other part of your body can be injured. The body responds to injury in predictable ways.

If you get a scratch on your arm, it will heal in a few days. If the tissue which lines the inside of one of your arteries is injured it will also heal. The body has well-developed, built-in mechanisms for wound healing. Problems with blood vessels arise if there are repeated injuries to the cells which line the inside of the vessels.

If the lining of one of the arteries in your body is injured, the healing process will begin. If the lining is reinjured before the healing process can be completed, this will, with time, lead to complications. The wall of the artery will start to thicken. Metabolic end-products will accumulate within the wall of the blood vessel. Fat and calcium will accumulate in the wall, causing the wall to thicken and harden. Hardening of the arteries—atherosclerosis—increases in most (but not all) individuals as they get older because of repeated injury to the cells which line the inside of the arteries.

The key to inhibiting the development of atherosclerosis—and the complications such as stroke and heart attack which follow its development—lies in inhibiting the processes which cause injury to the lining of the arteries.

What are some of the things that injure the lining of the arteries? The major ones are: (1) low blood levels of the "good" high-density lipoproteins (HDL); (2) high blood levels of the "bad" low-density lipoproteins (LDL); (3) the inhaling of toxic substances such as carbon monoxide or the ingestion of toxic substances such as heavy metals; and (4) high blood pressure. (High blood pressure injures the cells which line the inside of the ateries of the body *and* it causes the wall of the heart to thicken.) Reducing your body weight is helping you eliminate *three of the four* items listed above.

During the discussion of ways to inhibit aging of the muscular system, it was noted that muscles which are not properly exercised tend to get smaller and weaker. The heart is a muscle. Physical inactivity which does not regularly exercise the heart may cause the heart to lose some of its vigor. In addition, atherosclerosis compromises the flow of blood to the heart muscle. Both factors make the heart less able to perform at peak efficiency.

Blood clots may form in some of the arteries which supply blood to the heart. The clots form in sections of the arteries which have been narrowed by the buildup of plaque. When the clots obstruct the flow of blood to the heart muscle, the muscle cells begin to die and the heart becomes weaker. Dissolving the clots as soon as possible prevents damage to the heart muscle and, by doing so, saves lives. There is a drug called streptokinase, which if administered in the first few hours following a heart attack, can dissolve blood clots in the arteries which supply the heart muscle. Streptokinase dissolves clots, but it causes other problems such as excess bleeding and allergic reactions.

There is a new drug which, as of this writing, is being considered by an advisory panel to the Food and Drug Administration. The drug is called TPA (tissue plasminogen activator.) It has the potential of saving thousands of lives, since approximately 1,500 people in the U.S. die of heart attacks *each day*. TPA is produced by genetic engineering. (Genetic engineering involves the manipulation of genes for the controlled production or alteration of a biological molecule or product.) TPA dissolves clots but doesn't affect the body by causing excess bleeding the way streptokinase does. Because it is genetically engineered, it doesn't cause allergic reactions.

If some blood vessels supplying the heart muscles become "clogged," surgery may be required. In this type of surgery, blood vessels are borrowed from other parts of the body and attached above and below the clogged portion of the vessels which supply the heart. The blood is detoured around the clogged portion of the vessels. Since blood vessels which supply blood to the heart are called "coronary arteries," this type of surgery is known as a "coronary bypass."

Another method for relieving the obstruction in the coronary arteries is "transluminal coronary angioplasty." This is a long name for a procedure which involves placing a balloon-tipped catheter in the coronary artery and dilating the artery. The balloon "pushes out" the wall of the artery, making the opening larger so more blood can flow through the heart muscle.

You may wish to look upon aerobic exercise as a form of natural angioplasty—a "physiological" angioplasty. During exercise the vessels which supply blood to the heart dilate, and blood is pumped through them at a higher pressure than normal. This pushes on the wall of the dilated vessel. The opening through which blood flows is made larger so more blood can flow to the heart muscle.

If you participate in some type of regular activity, mentally visualize this "physiological angioplasty" taking place in the blood vessels of your heart as you exercise. *Hardening of the arteries is not an inevitable consequence of the aging process.* It is a disease! Atherosclerosis can be prevented and inhibited. Some scientists even believe that some phases of it are reversible.

If people could take a pill to protect themselves from heart disease, a lot of lives would be saved. Some individuals thought that just such a thing had become possible when the Omega-3 fish oils were discovered.

How does Omega-3 work? It affects certain cells in the blood, the platelets, in such a way that the blood doesn't clot as quickly as it normally would. Omega-3 does something else. It gives the body a favorable balance of substances called prostaglandins.

Prostaglandins are local hormones which affect smooth muscle action, the immune system, and other body functions. As a result of their effect on the amount and types of pros-taglandins in the body, the Omega-3s are protective against heart disease.

The results of a 20-year study of men in Holland confirmed this hypothesis (*New England Journal of Medicine,* May 9, 1985.) The men in the study who ate 7 to 11 ounces of cold-water fish each week had half the incidence of heart disease of men who did not eat fish. The study also showed that eating more than 7 to 11 ounces of fish each week did not offer additional protection. In other words, more was not better.

What about taking Omega-3 supplements? Obtaining Omega-3 through supplements can be costly and the supplements add calories to the diet. Also, since they can cause a person to bleed more easily—and may have other side effects—they should not be taken without the advice of a physician. If you wish to increase your intake of Omega-3, you can do it by eating foods which contain it.

You can get Omega-3 by eating cold-water fish such as salmon and mackerel. (Remember 7 to 11 ounces a week is all you need.) If you don't particularly care for fish, you can get Omega-3 from soybeans, ordinary beans, and walnuts.

Omega-3 is not a cure-all for heart and blood vessel disease. It is desirable that you have some in your diet, but improving the health of your heart and blood vessels requires attention to additional factors such as exercise, weight control, and good nutrition in general. Good cardiovascular fitness comes from good health practices, not from a capsule. The heart and blood vessels were built to last. They have lasted for more than 100 years in thousands of people, and every day we learn something new about how to care for them.

What can be done to inhibit the aging process of the cardiovascular system? Five important ways are listed below: (1) Increase the level of the "good" HDL in your blood. You are currently doing this by lowering your body weight. You are also doing it if you are engaging in a regular program of exercise.

(2) Reduce the level of the "bad" LDL in your blood. You are currently doing this by lowering your body weight. You are also doing this if you have reduced your intake of saturated fats and cholesterol-containing foods.

(3) Stimulate your cardiovascular system with daily exercise. If the heart muscle is exercised properly, it will maintain its vigor for a longer period of time.

(4) Avoid inhaling or ingesting toxic substances.

(5) Reduce your blood pressure if it is high. You are currently doing this by lowering your body weight. *Take steps to keep your blood pressure at a normal level even if some medication is required.*

Note: If you want to know how much your blood cholesterol level is changing as your weight decreases, you may be interested in a new method which has been developed to determine blood cholesterol. The method takes just a few minutes of time and requires only a drop of blood. Until now, blood had to be drawn from a vein and subjected to involved laboratory tests in order to determine the amount of cholesterol in it.

This new method will make it possible to screen large numbers of people for high blood cholesterol. That could play a significant role in reducing the incidence of heart and blood vessel disease in the U.S. People are more inclined to take steps to lower their blood cholesterol levels if they know what it is, if they know it is too high, and if they know how to lower it.

Thousands of people live for more than 100 years. That is an indication that, with proper care, the cardiovascular system is quite capable of functioning for prolonged periods of time.

Things to do during Week Twenty-Five: If you go out to eat or to visit relatives and friends, you can continue to use this method of resetting your body weight to a new level. Continue to follow the steps. Say, "I'm full" and "Do I have to eat it all?" to yourself at the appropriate times. Use the visualizations.

Tell yourself that you are "slim and trim" and that you "weigh _____ pounds" when you see your reflection. Later when you have the opportunity, you can record your points and make comments if appropriate.

If possible read *something* from this book even when you go to visit friends and relatives.

WEEK TWENTY-SIX

Comments: Ways to prevent the premature aging of the respiratory system, nervous system, urinary system and reproductive system will be considered this week.

Respiratory System. How can one prevent premature aging of the respiratory system? The answers to that one are simple: (1) Use it. (2) Don't injure it. The phrase "use it or lose it" can be appropriately applied to the respiratory system. If you wish to maintain the integrity, viability, and vigor of your respiratory system, you must "use it."

As an individual gets older, the airways and the air sacs in the lungs lose some of their elasticity. That might cause some small reduction in the amount of air that a person can breathe in and out, but there are other factors. During normal respiration, the diaphragm (the muscle beneath the rib cage) contracts to pull air into the lungs. If you take a very deep breath, the diaphragm contracts more vigorously. In addition, the muscles of the rib cage contract to raise the rib cage. This pulls even more air into the lungs. If these muscles become weaker, the amount of air that can be breathed in and out will be reduced.

The diaphragm becomes weaker and the walls of the chest become more rigid with age. Exercising the diaphragm can, as with any muscle, maintain its strength for a longer period of time. Taking deep breaths daily can maintain the full range of motion of the joints of the rib cage and prevent the rib cage from becoming rigid.

There are small air sacs in the lungs. Inhaling toxic substances such as smoke, carbon monoxide, auto exhaust, emissions, industrial pollutants, and particles of matter such as coal dust and asbestos causes these sacs to rupture. Once ruptured they don't "grow back" even if you quit inhaling substances which injure them. If a large number of air sacs rupture, the volume of air which can be breathed into and out of the lungs is reduced. A severe reduction in the number of air sacs in the lungs as a result of their rupturing is called emphysema. Emphysema can progress to the point that an individual may actually die of air hunger while under an oxygen tent. In such individuals there is just not enough lung tissue left for the transfer of gases between the air and the blood.

People sometimes think that the most dangerous effect of cigarette smoking is lung cancer. Lung cancer is a devastating disease to the person who has it, but smoking affects you even if you don't get lung cancer. Perhaps the most serious effect of cigarette smoking on the population in general is that it speeds up the rate of hardening of the arteries. That significantly reduces the life expectancy of people in the United States. Some scientists believe that smoking reduces the life expectancy of individuals by six to eight years.

Some people believe that they can either smoke and keep

their weight down, or not smoke and gain weight. That isn't really the case. The weight that they gain after they stop smoking is usually temporary. It is worth putting up with a transient increase in body weight to increase life expectancy by six to eight years. (Besides, you now have a method for controlling your weight.)

When you quit smoking, a substance (nicotine) which your body is accustomed to having begins to be cleared out of your body. When that happens, your body sends the message that, "you had better get it or you won't survive." Objectively, people know that they don't need nicotine to survive, so they substitute food in an attempt to satisfy the craving. They gain weight until the nicotine is cleared from their body. When the craving goes away they usually stop overeating.

Smoking decreases the respiratory function as does the inhaling of other toxic substances. Often when we see that there is a reduction in respiratory function, we mistakenly attribute it to the aging process when, in reality, it is a reduction in function because of disuse and/or injury.

How can the aging process of the respiratory system be inhibited? There are two important ways:

(1) Taking large breaths—as large as possible—whether by purposeful breathing or as a result of physical activity, will exercise the diaphragm and the muscles of the chest wall. Taking breaths will give full range of motion to the joints of the chest wall. It is important that this be done *each day*.

(2) A decrease in respiratory function can be avoided by not inhaling toxic substances.

If you breathe in as much air as you can, then exhale as much air as you can, that volume of air is called the vital capacity. The vital capacity may decrease by as much as 35 to 40 percent by the time a person reaches the age of 70. But it *need not* decrease that much! Daily, deep vigorous breathing will inhibit the early reduction of your vital capacity. Losing weight will allow you to breathe larger volumes of air in and out of your lungs because the excess weight doesn't restrict the movement of the diaphragm.

Nervous System. Neurologists tell us that we lose nerve cells as we grow older. Nerve cells are lost daily, but millions must be lost before there is severe compromise of function of the nervous system. As the nerve cells are lost, there is a decrease in the ability to send impulses to and from the brain and from place to place within the brain. With advancing age, recent memory may be affected—we can remember the name of our first grade teacher but not what we had for lunch yesterday.

It is a known fact that many individuals remain mentally alert and creative after they are well into their years. Why? How is it possible to postpone the effects of aging on the nervous system? Why does premature aging of the nervous system seem to happen to some people and not to others?

The maintenance of a good blood supply and a good oxygen supply to the brain is probably one of the most important factors. The brain will have a good blood supply and a good oxygen supply if the cardiovascular system and the respiratory system are functioning properly. The inhibition of the aging process of the respiratory system was discussed above and the inhibition of the aging process of the cardiovascular system was discussed during WEEK TWENTY-FIVE. A reduced oxygen supply—it is called "hypoxia"—causes injury and death to brain cells quicker than it causes injury and death to most other cells of the body. Sometimes we might think that loss of mental alertness in an individual was caused by age, when it really was caused by poor circulation of blood.

A ready supply of nutrients is also essential to the continued good health of nerve cells. Harmful agents such as carbon monoxide and other toxic substances injure and kill nerve cells just as they injure and kill other cells of the body.

Some individuals claim that the continued, energetic use of nerve cells helps maintain the cells' vigor, integrity and length of life. (That makes sense—it works for other cells of the body.) They cite as examples a long list of creative individuals—artists, writers, scientists, executives, entertainers and others—who live for a very long time and remain creative for as long as they live. Whether that claim is true or not, it *is* a fact of life that it is possible to live to a very old age while remaining creative and mentally alert.

The things that can be done to help prevent premature aging of the nervous system are given below. There is a question mark beside the fourth item listed. While it is important to exercise the nerve cells, exercise is a "maybe" as far as inhibiting the aging process of the nervous system is concerned. How can you exercise nerve cells? Whenever you play a musical instrument, plan a future event, learn something new, or do anything creative, you are exercising nerve cells by sending impulses across them. It may be that your nerve cells will remain viable longer if they are exercised regularly.

(1) Work toward maintaining a good blood and oxygen supply to the nervous system. This can be done by keeping the respiratory and cardiovascular systems healthy.

(2) Eat nutritious foods.

(3) Avoid inhaling or ingesting toxic substances.

(4) Exercise the nerve cells by continuing to use them vigorously.(?)

Urinary System. By the time an individual reaches the age of 70, the number of filtering units in the kidney (nephrons) may be reduced by as much as one-half. This poses no particular problem since it is possible to lead quite a normal life as long as 35 to 40 percent of the nephrons are functional. That is comforting to know, but we still want to lose as few of our nephrons as possible as we get older.

How can we keep from losing more nephrons than we should as we get older? Such precautions as: (1) a proper diet; (2) the ingestion of liquids that are beneficial and the avoidance of those that are harmful to the kidney; (3) the avoidance of hazardous agents; (4) the avoidance of infectious diseases (and getting immediate treatment if contracted); and (5) immediate attention to kidney and urinary tract problems; will all help to prevent an unnecessary loss of nephrons with age.

The kidneys are capable of functioning quite well for prolonged periods of time. Since it is not possible to live without kidneys (unless one is being dialyzed with a kidney machine), it follows that individuals who live to be 90 or 100 years of age have an adequate number of nephrons. You can, too.

Reproductive System. With advancing age, there is a decrease in fertility in both males and females. The production of estrogens and progesterone in the female and of testosterone in the male decreases. The number of sperm cells is reduced, although abundant sperm cells may be found even in old age.

Many individuals remain sexually active after they are old. Their ability to do so seems more related to their general physical and mental health than to their age. Thus following the steps outlined during the past five weeks for inhibiting the aging process of the other systems of the body will enhance one's ability to remain sexually active into old age.

Note: While the material for this week was being written, this author had occasion to talk to: (1) a 74-year-old man who continues to work ten hours a day—he lifts and moves objects weighing 100 pounds and more just as he has always done; (2) an 84-year-old man who gave up yacht racing three years ago because of some loss of vision in one eye and some "circulation problems" in one leg—he continues to be active and spends a lot of time traveling; (3) a 96-year old woman whose vision is good but who needs glasses to read. She has "no trouble eating" but can't get about like she used to because of "knee joint problems."

Chapter 9

How Food Intake Affects Life Expectancy and Life Span
(Weeks 27–28)

WEEK TWENTY-SEVEN

Comments: The comments of this week will center initially on life *expectancy* and then a discussion of life *span* will follow.

What is the difference between life *expectancy* and life *span*? Basically, life *expectancy* is the length of time we can expect to live, considering the number of hazards we encounter every day. In other words it can be thought of as our "chances of survival," or our "odds" for making it for a given period of time. Life *expectancy* is determined by the number of dangerous things we overcome or avoid. Life *span* is determined by our "aging clock." The "aging clocks" of the turtle, the human and the laboratory rat are different. If everything works perfectly for all three during their respective lives, the turtle will live for 200 years, the human will live for 100 years and the laboratory rat will live for three years. Their "aging clocks" are different, so their life spans are different. (More about life span later.)

Life Expectancy. The life expectancy of people living in the United States has passed 70 years and is moving toward 80 years. If we use the interventions which are currently available to us, it is possible that we will see the bulk of humans living, in good health, for 90 years and more.

Can something be done to increase the human life expectancy? Certainly! You are increasing yours now by losing weight! Humans die because of diseases and accidents. Something can be done about both. More specifically, the vast majority of humans die as a result of (1) heart and blood vessel diseases, (2) cancer, and (3) accidents.

Heart and blood vessel diseases alone account for 48 percent of the deaths in the United States! Hardening of the arteries, heart attack, stroke, and high blood pressure are not just "inevitable consequences of the aging process." They don't have to occur. They are diseases, and diseases have preventions and cures. (Not all of the preventions and cures for all diseases have been found yet, but in my opinion, they will be.)

You now know how to avoid bringing on premature aging of the cardiovascular system. By losing weight you are changing the lipid (fat) profile in your blood so that the HDL is increasing and the LDL is decreasing. Your blood pressure is coming down. Your heart is not having to work as hard as it had been working. Since you are moving your weight to a new level, you are practicing preventive medicine. You are accepting a responsibility for your own health by adopting a new, healthier lifestyle.

Years ago people apparently had a different view of things. They went about doing pretty much as they pleased with respect to the way they took care of themselves. Then when things started to break down and come apart, they would go to see their doctor and say in effect, "Okay Doc, here I am. Fix me up." No wonder life expectancy was so short then! There was very little good information available to individuals on how to take care of themselves. To further complicate things, physicians of the time had fewer means at their disposal with which to "fix up" their patients.

You are reducing your risk of cancer (and thus increasing your life expectancy) by losing weight. The relationship between mortality from cancer (and other diseases) and variation in weight among 750,000 men and women selected from the general population has been examined (Lew and Garfinkel, 1979). Cancer mortality was significantly elevated in both sexes among those who were 40 percent or more overweight. The excess mortality in men resulted from cancer of the digestive system (colon and rectum). In women the excess mortality resulted from cancer of the gall bladder, breast, cervix, and ovary.

Studies in experimental animals have shown that caloric restriction inhibits the development and growth of certain tumors. Reducing the level of dietary fat reduces the rate of growth of skin tumors and breast tumors (but not of lung tumors) in experimental animals. In addition, studies have shown that animals on restricted diets develop fewer tumors in general. Their life expectancy exceeds that of animals which are fed all the food they want whenever they want it. To say it another way, a reduction in total food intake decreases the age-specific incidence of cancer in animals and increases their life expectancy.

Will you be less likely to get cancer if you eat certain types of foods? The top scientists in the field think so. They believe that many cancer deaths in this country can be avoided if we make some changes in our eating habits. The American Institute of Cancer Research (AICR), Washington, D.C., 20069, has recently published some dietary guidelines for lowering cancer risks. In summary, these common-sense guidelines stress a few basic things: They recommend that the intake of saturated and unsaturated fat be lowered from the current average of approximately 40 percent to a level of 30 percent of total calories. They recommend that the consumption of fruits, vegetables, and whole-grain cereals be increased. They urge moderation in the consumption of salt-cured, smoked and charcoal-broiled foods, and moderation in the consumption of alcoholic beverages. Those recommendations are simple and straightforward. There is data to back up claims that nutrition of this type can lower your chances of getting cancer!

Some diets have been found to enhance the growth of cancer in experimental animals and others have been found to inhibit the growth of chemically caused cancers. Studies such as these led investigators to examine the role of nutrition in cancer in humans. That is the way the above guidelines evolved.

For example, in such studies, it was found that there is a lower incidence of breast cancer and colon cancer in population groups whose diets are low in fats. Americans are switching from saturated fats to unsaturated fats. That might lower serum cholesterol levels and make one less likely to get heart disease. Lowering the *total* fat intake will make one less likely to get certain types of cancer.

There is more good news relative to cancer and nutrition. According to the AICR, certain nutrients and other food constituents such as vitamins A, C, and E, selenium, and dietary fiber may be anticancer substances. The AICR recommends that these substances be consumed *at levels found in a balanced diet.* (More is not always better. Nutritional excesses may be related to chronic diseases.) Vitamin A is associated with lower risk of most cancers, vitamin C is associated with reduced risks of cancers of the stomach and esophagus, and vitamin E has been shown to protect against cancer in some experimental animals. The data on vitamin E in humans is only preliminary at this time. The cancer mortality rates are higher in areas where selenium consumption is low and vice versa.

Where are the above substances found? Vitamin A is found in dark green and deep yellow vegetables; vitamin C is found in fruits; vitamin E is found in whole-grain cereals, soybeans and leafy greens; selenium is found in bran, tuna fish, and tomatoes; and dietary fiber is found in vegetables, fruits, and whole grains.

Better methods of detecting and treating cancer are rapidly becoming available. Here is an example of each: A simple blood test, done with nuclear magnetic resonance spectroscopy and requiring only a few minutes, holds the promise of detecting almost any type of cancer (Fossel, *New England Journal of Medicine,* 1986). Many cancers which are detected early are treatable. With regard to treatment, radioactive antibodies, produced with the tools of genetic engineering and nuclear medicine, will soon be tested on patients with colon cancer and later perhaps on patients with lung, skin, and other types of cancer. These antibodies hit the tumor and leave the rest of the body alone. These are just two examples of the types of detection and treatment which are currently being investigated.

You are reducing your risk of cancer by moving your weight to a new level. Enormous strides have been made in finding better methods of prevention, detection and treatment of cancer. The mechanisms which cause cancer are better understood than ever before. Some cancers which were not treatable years ago are now treatable and curable. In time others will be also. Exciting new information is forthcoming.

Another major cause of deaths is accidents. Accidents claim thousands of lives each year. Concern for the loss of human lives—not to mention the billions of dollars of property damage—has directed our attention to finding methods of preventing accidents in the home, on the road and in the industrial setting. You see safety devices all about you. The efforts are working.

Okay, so heart and blood vessel disease, cancer, and accidents do cause the vast majority of deaths in the United States. Something can, and is, being done about all three. What about the other causes of death? There are a multitude of other causes of death such as brain diseases, kidney diseases, acquired immune deficiency syndrome (AIDS), and rare genetic disorders. Is something being done about them? Yes. Methods for the prevention, treatment and cure of virtually every cause of death are being vigorously studied. That is the reason our life expectancy has passed 70 years and is moving toward 80 years. That is the reason humans are living longer—in good health—than ever before.

You are moving your life expectancy nearer to your life span. Suppose, just suppose, that everything worked perfectly for all of us. Suppose that our life expectancy moved all the way *to* our life span. (The figure 100 years has been used in our discussion of life span but the human life span is probably somewhere around 110 years.) If our life expectancy moves *to* our life span, is that the end of the story? Is it impossible to adjust Mother Nature's "aging clock?" The answer is going to startle you! Let us turn our attention to the subject of life span.

Life Span. It is common knowledge that different animal species live for different lengths of time. The reason is that their "aging clocks" are set differently. Animals, humans included, don't just "get old and die." After they are born, they mature, then grow old and die because it is a *programmed change!* If aging "just happened" with the passing of time, then all animals would live the same length of time; they would have the same life span; and they would all age at the same rate. But they don't all age at the same rate. All animals don't have the same life span.

In the human, and presumably in other animal species, if the programmed aging mechanism is either absent or not functioning properly, there is a dramatic change in the rate of aging. The entire aging process may take place in a fraction of the time that would normally be required.

You have probably seen children on television or in the newspapers who have the syndrome known as "progeria." Progeria is a premature senility syndrome. Children who have

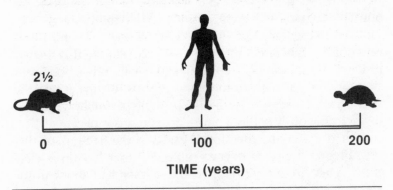

Figure 7. This figure graphically illustrates the life spans of the laboratory rat, the human, and the Galapagos tortoise. Life span differences are due to the fact that their "aging clocks" do not operate at the same speed.

it develop normally during the first year. That first year of normal development is followed by retardation of growth and a rapidly developing senile appearance. There is loss of hair, wrinkling of the skin and other obvious signs of aging. The *entire aging process* occurs while the individuals are still young! They grow old and many die before they reach an age when they should be in early puberty. Why? Their "aging clock" is either absent or not functioning properly.

Where is the "aging clock" located? How does it work? The exact way the "aging clock" works in not completely understood at this time. There are several theories about its location and the way it controls aging. Let us examine some of the theories regarding the structure and function of the "controller of aging" in the body.

One theory of aging is that the cells of the body can only divide so many times. There is strong evidence for this theory because cells taken from the body and grown outside the body divide only a limited number of times and then stop. If they are taken from an older person, they divide fewer times than do similar cells taken from a younger person. If they are taken from an animal with a short life span, they divide fewer times than if they are taken from an animal with a long life span. According to this theory, the stopping of cell division is a normal programmed event. Some cells of the body are not replaced if they are lost. Heart cells, muscle cells and nerve cells don't regenerate if they are lost. According to this theory, losing cells that can't be replaced, and having other body cells stop dividing is a part of the aging process. But what tells the cells when to stop dividing? What tells them how fast to divide? Obviously some "controller" is responsible.

A theory of aging mentioned earlier is the free-radical theory. Free radicals are oxygen molecules that have free electrons. They are highly reactive and as they flail about inside and outside the cells of the body, they weaken the protein of the cells and may destroy the cells. With time, cells become more rigid and their surface changes, so it is more difficult for them to get nutrients in and waste materials out. (As noted earlier, substances such as vitamin C, vitamin E and selenium inhibit the formation of free radicals.) Free radical formation is probably not a complete answer to the aging process and to life span. Again, there must be an overall "controller" of life span because of the extreme differences seen in the life spans of animals of different species. If the rate of free radical formation controlled the aging process and life span, then most animals would have essentially the same life span.

Some who study the aging process believe that changes in the immune system are responsible for the aging process. The immune system manufactures antibodies to protect us against foreign invaders. (Recall from earlier discussions that stress adversely affects the immune system.) According to the immune theory of aging, as the surface of the cells of the body changes, the immune system turns against its own cells. In other words, the more the surface of the cell changes, the more rapidly the immune system forms antibodies to attack the body's own cells. This may be a partial answer, but the question arises as to what controls the speed of the process. Why do cell surfaces change faster in some animals than in others? Why does the immune system turn against its own cells faster in some animals than in others? This brings up the question once again as to the identity of the overall "controller" of life span.

Others who study the aging process believe that at a certain time in life, a hormone is released into the body which starts the aging process. According to this hypothesis, the syndrome "progeria" could be explained by the fact that an aging hormone is released at a very early age. Also, according to the theory, the fact that different animal species have different life spans could be explained by the fact that the hormone is released earlier in some animals than in others.

Another possibility is that there is an as yet unidentified "life" hormone. It might well come from the hypothalamus. There are a multitude of substances which are released from the hypothalamus, substances which control glands and other body functions. According to this theory of aging, the level of this "life" hormone in the body is high in the early years. The level of the hormone in the body gradually decreases with time, producing the effects of aging. If it decreases faster in some species, the life span will be short. If it decreases more slowly in other species, the life span will be long. This hormone (or substance) could be a polypeptide.

A *polypeptide* is formed when several organic acid molecules are linked together. Many hormones and very active substances in the body are polypeptides, and a number of them are produced by the hypothalamus. (The endorphins which were discussed during WEEK FIFTEEN are polypeptides.) Thus the possibility that there is such a "controller of aging" which is a polypeptide and which is produced by the hypothalamus is an attractive hypothesis. The possible existence of such a substance raises some exciting questions. Can the substance be identified? Can its structure be determined? Can the substance be made synthetically?

It is stimulating to think about the possibilities which could result from the identification of a "life hormone." That has not been accomplished at this time, although some studies regarding manipulation of life span have been done. They will be discussed next week.

Things to do during Week Twenty-Seven: Follow all of the steps. Record your points daily. When appropriate, record your comments also.

WEEK TWENTY-EIGHT

Comments: The *life span* of experimental animals can be *increased* by reducing their food intake! It doesn't matter if the reduction in food intake is started when they are weaned or if it is started after they become adults. The result is the same: the life span increases!

Years ago one investigator (McCay, 1934) had the idea that if he could keep animals from maturing, he could increase their life span. He thought that all of the aging processes in animals occurred after they reach maturity. He tried to keep his animals from maturing by feeding them less food. He wanted to keep them the size they were when they were weaned. He was not able to do that and he was not able to keep them from reaching maturity, but he did made an interesting discovery. In conducting his experiments, he significantly reduced the animals' food intake. By doing so he caused some of them to live a very long time. In other words, he increased their life span. He thought it was because he was able to delay their maturing, but the cause was actually the food restriction. It was later shown that food restriction which is started after animals become adults will also increase the life span.

Remember the earlier discussions about how the different systems of the body change with time? The muscular system, the nervous system, and the other systems of the body progressively change as individuals get older. Recently it was shown that reducing the food intake not only increases the life span, it also inhibits a number of the basic aging processes of the different systems of the body. Reducing the food intake inhibits many of the *natural* changes that take place as animals age. Reducing food intake delays the onset and slows the development of age-related *diseases*.

One carefully designed study strikingly demonstrated this relationship. Two groups of laboratory rats were used, with 115 animals in each group. They were all raised in a protected environment. The rats in the first group were fed *ad libitum*. (That is, they were fed as much food as they wanted whenever they wanted it throughout their lives.) The amount of food that they ate was measured. The food intake of the second group of animals was restricted; they were given 60 percent of the amount of food that the first group ate. Both groups of animals were simply allowed to grow old and die.

The group of animals which *ate less food* had a *longer life span!* When the very last animal in the group on the high food intake died, approximately 70 percent of all of the animals on reduced food intake were still alive! The average length of life of the animals on the high food intake was approximately 700 days. The average length of life of the animals whose food intake was reduced was 986 days. Food restriction increased their life span by approximately 40 percent.

A number of changes occur in different systems of the body as individuals get older. These changes and some ways to inhibit them have already been discussed. Most of the age-related changes in the body systems of the animals in the experiments described above were either slowed or prevented by food restriction. Here is something—food restriction—which *actually increases life span*. Medicine and technology have helped increase our life *expectancy*. Now here is evidence to indicate that the life span itself can be changed.

In the experiments described above, the food restriction increased the life span of the animals. How did it do that? Probably by prolonging the life span of all of the different systems in their body. For example:

(1) The blood cholesterol levels increase with age in this particular type of animal. Restricting the food intake almost totally prevented the increase in blood cholesterol with age.

(2) As the animals on the high food intake got older, the level of a particular type of hormone in their blood increased. The hormone is called calcitonin. It lowers the amount of calcium in the blood. It is not desirable to have the blood level of calcitonin increase. Food restriction markedly reduced the increase in the blood level of calcitonin as the animals got older.

(3) Muscle cells are lost as animals get order. The loss of muscle mass was delayed by food restriction, as was the loss of muscle function.

(4) There is a particular type of muscle in the body called smooth muscle. It is found in the walls of the intestine, in the blood vessels, and in other places. Muscle cells of this type are also lost with age. Food restriction inhibited the age-related changes in the smooth muscle cells.

(5) As animals, humans included, get older, the bones age.

Bone mass is lost. The loss of bone mass was delayed by food restriction.

(6) There are certain types of receptors in the brain which are lost as animals get older. The loss of these receptors was delayed by food restriction.

All of the other systems in the body were probably affected in a similar fashion. The food restriction inhibited the effects normally associated with aging.

One theory of aging is that changes in the immune system are responsible for the aging process. It is believed that the immune system turns against its own cells. As time passes, the surface of the cells of the body changes and the immune system forms antibodies to attack the body's own cells. The aging of the immune system is delayed by food restriction. The autoimmunity which occurs in mice as they get older is delayed by food restriction.

The hormones of the body act on particular cells of the body called target cells. The target cells tend to become less responsive with age. Food restriction delays that change. The target cells of the food-restricted animals continued to be responsive for a longer period of time.

It is clear that food restriction made the animals live longer because it increased the "life span" of all of their body systems. Remember that "life span" is a programmed event. The food restriction somehow interfered with that program.

One investigator (Yu, 1984) studied the effects of reduced food intake on *diseases* that develop in animals as they get older. In the animals which he studied, chronic nephropathy (kidney diseases) occurred in nearly all of the animals as they got older. (In that respect it is similar to hardening of the arteries, a disease which occurs in almost all humans as they get older.) Food restriction so successfully slowed the development of chronic nephropathy in the animals that almost none of them (less than three percent) had the disease. Of the group with high food intake, 72 percent had the disease.

Another disease which occurred in the animals studied by Yu was cardiomyopathy, a disease of the heart muscle. Reduced food intake delayed the development of cardiomyopathy. Reduced food intake also significantly delayed the development of cancers in the animals.

All of the above information clearly demonstrates the very broad way in which food restriction affects changes that occur with age. Virtually everything in the body is affected. The importance of the observation is that food restriction is likely getting at the very heart of the aging process. That is, *it is slowing the "aging clock."* Food restriction apparently slows the "aging clock" and that, in turn, slows the aging of all of the systems of the body. By slowing the aging of all of the systems of the body, the life span is increased. In other words, food restriction retards a basic aging process in the experimental animal.

Yu's elegant studies strike the very nucleus of the mystery of *life span*. Reduced food intake caused the seemingly unstoppable aging process to pause; caused it to pause long enough to extend the *life span* of the animals he studied by more than 30 percent. How? Did it interfere with the metabolic machinery of aging, or did it elicit the release of a "regulating" substance which maintained the viability of the life processes? Both possibilities are plausible, both are significant, and both deserve further study.

It's remarkable that reduced food intake interferes with the basic aging process of *all* of the systems of the body and not with just one or two systems. Perhaps it decreases the rate of aging by changing the metabolism of the different systems of the body. A more appealing hypothesis is that reduced food intake promotes the continued existence of a "life" hormone. If that is the case, then it is very likely that stimuli other than reduced food intake can cause the body to continue producing the "life" hormone for a longer period of time and, by doing so, increase the life span.

What other types of stimuli could do that? Some possibilities are intense mental activity, intense physical activity, or altered light-dark cycles.

Suppose the "life" hormone is a compound from the family

of polypeptides which originate in the hypothalamus. Polypeptides from the hypothalamus perform a number of body regulatory functions. It seems reasonable that the hormone which determines the overall rate of aging should come from the hypothalamus.

Food restriction stimulates the release of polypeptides (endorphins) from the hypothalamus. Aerobic exercise stimulates the release of polypeptides (endorphins) from the hypothalamus. Maybe intense mental activity and changes in the light-dark cycle also stimulate the release of polypeptides.

Since food restriction, aerobic activity, and other stimuli cause the release of polypeptides from the hypothalamus, perhaps something else happens. Perhaps concomitant with the release of those polypeptides, the polypeptide which is the "regulator" of, and which prolongs life span is "dragged out" along with the other polypeptides. Speculation? Maybe. But food restriction does increase life span in the experimental animal. That is a proven fact!

Can life span be increased? Yes. Life span has been increased in the experimental animal. The implication is that more knowledge in this area might lead to interventions for adjusting the life span of other animals, including humans.

Things to do during Week Twenty-Eight: Do not think in terms of consciously restricting your food intake. Follow all of the steps. Record your points daily. When appropriate, record your comments also.

Chapter 10

Look at You Now!
(Weeks 29–30 and Beyond)

WEEK TWENTY-NINE

Comments: You are losing weight. It is obvious. You are changing. It is only natural that others are going to ask you how you are doing it. *Make it a special project to help someone through the program.* That will do two things. First, that will help someone else lose weight. Second, the continued repetition will help to insure that your weight control center is more permanently set. By the time the person you are helping reaches WEEK THIRTY, you will have gone through a cycle of more than a year. You will have gone through all of the seasons, the holidays, vacations, and gatherings with family and friends. You will know that the resetting process has continued through all of that time.

While you are helping someone with this program, continue on your own program of body weight adjustment. Whether you are helping someone with this program or simply sharing the information as the two of you progress through it together, you may find the following information helpful in answering questions which may arise.

During WEEK TEN it was mentioned that some "miracle cures" for obesity would be mentioned at a later time. There is a reason for waiting until this particular time to mention some additional cures. Anyone interested in adjusting his body weight—anyone you help—will be concerned about other types of "cures." He will want to know if this or that "cure" works. He will want to know if something works better or if it works faster than what he is now doing. You know that all of the "cures" basically involve overriding the appestat or fooling the appestat. (Some do neither and are fraudulent.) If you have specific information about some of the "cures" for obesity which are on the market, you will be better able to help someone with the program. You will be better able to answer his questions.

There are a multitude of fad diets, pills, potions, and devices which are available if you are willing to pay the going price for them. There are wraps to melt it off, belts to work it off, and foods and magic pills to "burn it off." There are electrical devices to "exercise" it off. (The devices are useful to the physical therapist, but useless for reducing body weight.) There are a multitude of "secret" and "magic" formulas. Some are moderately costly, some are expensive, and some are exorbitant. It is beyond the scope of this book to mention all of them, but it is important to mention some of the more popular ones.

You now know how to set your weight to a new level. There is nothing "magic" or "secret" about it. During the time the material for this week was being written, no fewer that four "new," wonderful diets came across my desk. Three of them were simply variations of a basic, safe 1200-calorie, balanced diet. The other was a diet that guaranteed 20 pounds of weight loss in 14 days and was downright dangerous. It cautioned individuals "not to stay on this diet more than 14 days at a time." That was good advice. Better advice would have been not to get on the diet at all. The diet consisted essentially of protein plus low-calorie foods such as celery, cucumbers, cabbage, and grapefruit. It recommended that individuals consume only 400 to 500 calories a day. The calories would come almost totally from protein. That would cause fat deposits in the body to be broken down for energy more quickly than the body could use them. Compounds called ketone bodies would form and be excreted in the urine. A person would lose some body water in the process. His body would get the energy it required from the muscles and other major organs. The metabolic rate would be slowed, setting the body up to regain the weight that was lost (plus some extra weight) as soon as normal eating was resumed. The diet is *dangerous*.

The extent to which we search for a "magic potion" for weight loss is exemplified by a recent flyer which carried the message that consuming large quantities of water is the answer to permanent weight loss. It is true that the body does require adequate fluids. It is also true that some loss of appetite may accompany increased consumption of water, but that does not render water a panacea for weight control.

When "new," wonderful diets come to your attention, ask yourself two questions: (1) Are they *safe* and *effective*? (2) Would it be reasonable to expect a person to stay on them for the remainder of his/her life?

Suits, wraps, belts and gels that cause you to "sweat it off" produce a temporary loss of weight. Weight is lost because water is lost. When one drinks fluid, the weight is regained.

Glucomannan is a substance which has been promoted as an Oriental weight loss secret. It is a fiber source that comes from Konjac root. When eaten it creates a feeling of fullness just as do carrots, lettuce, apples, and other bulky foods.

Another substance which has been promoted as a weight loss agent is human chrionic gonadotropin (HCG). HCG is a legitimate hormone which is used by obstetricians and gynecologists to treat reproductive problems. The American Medical Association has stated that the substance, while valuable in treating reproductive problems, is useless for weight loss.

In the past, amphetamines have been used to promote weight loss. But they are addicting and have undesirable effects on the heart and on the nervous system. They would be harmful to one's health if used for a prolonged period of time. They should not be used for weight loss.

There are several over-the-counter diet pills. Phenylpropanolamine (PPA) is the active substance in many of them. PPA appears to be safe for some, but it should not be taken by anyone who has high blood pressure, gout, thyroid problems, diabetes, or kidney problems. A 1986 research report to the American Society of Pharmacology and Experimental Therapeutics by R. Quirk and associates indicates that PPA may occasionally cause hypertension, insomnia, heart palpitations, psychotic reactions, and headaches. Based on those observations, one has to question whether or not it would be advisable even for a healthy person to take PPA for an extended period of time.

Another ingredient in over-the-counter candies and gums is benzocaine. Benzocaine is said to numb the sense of taste. One would have to question the advisability of taking this substance forever—or, for that matter, whether numbing the sense of taste could override the powerful weight control system permanently. (If some substance does prove to be an aid in weight loss and *can't be taken forever,* then one runs the risk of entering into a cycle of weight loss with rebound weight gain when normal eating is resumed. Also, more difficulty will be experienced by the individual the next time a diet or magic pill is used to lose weight.)

Claims have been made that DHEA—its chemical name is dehydroepiandrosterone—will promote weight loss in an individual. DHEA is a breakdown product of hormones obtained from human urine. DHEA is normally excreted from the body. It is not known what effect this substance might have on the body when it is put back into the body in concentrated form. Data does not seem to exist to substantiate claims that it will cause weight loss.

Starch blockers are said to block the absorption of carbohydrates. These claims have not been proven. There have been reports of adverse gastrointestinal effects as a result of using the starch blockers. They are unapproved new drugs and have been declared illegal.

Spirulina, another agent promoted as a weight-loss substance, is derived from algae. It can be legally sold if it is labeled as a food. It supposedly contains an appetite suppressant called phenylalanine, but it has not been scientifically proven that phenylalanine is an appetite suppressant.

If someone mentions pills which "burn fat" while you sleep, they are probably referring to pills which contain arginine and ornithine. They supposedly cause you to burn fat by stimulating hormone production, particularly growth hormone. If this claim is true, they would be dangerous, because they could cause the level of hormones in the blood to increase. This would adversely affect many of the body's systems and the body's overall metabolism.

(Some of the above information was taken from the Department of Health and Human Services Publication No. 85-1116.) This publication and other publications regarding food, nutrition and exercise may be obtained free of charge by writing Consumer Information Center, P.O. Box 100, Pueblo, CO 81002.)

Chances are that almost anyone who is overweight will tell you that he has lost weight at one time or another. If you are helping such a person and if you ask, "What happened?", he will invariably say, "I gained it back." Losing weight and then gaining it back often makes people think that they don't have willpower. They think that there is some kind of flaw in their character because they are overweight and other people are not. Now you know why some people are overweight and others aren't: their appestats are set at different levels. It has nothing to do with willpower, or strength of character, or determination, or *anything* other than having appestats set at different levels.

Suppose you randomly selected 100 overweight people who wanted to lose weight. Then you gave all of them a well-balanced, 1200 calorie diet. How many of them do you think would *lose all of the weight they wanted to lose*? Would you believe that only about ten out of the 100 would? Of the ten who lost all of the weight they wanted to lose, only two would keep the weight off permanently. (If a person keeps weight off for one to two years, that is considered "permanent" by many who study body weight control.) That is a pretty grim statistic, isn't it? Only *two people* out of the 100 people you randomly selected would lose all of the weight they wanted to lose *and* keep it off for one to two years. (Even those two probably can't override their weight control center for the *rest of their lives!*) That is the reason it is not uncommon to talk to someone who has lost weight then "gained it back." Many people try to lose weight. A recent newspaper headline (*U.S.A. Today* 8/11/86) proclaimed, "One in three on diet."

Since you are mentally adjusting your body weight, this is a method you can continue to use wherever you are. You can use it if you fly into an airport, have a layover and need to eat a bite. You can use it if you go on vacation to the mountains, or to the seashore, or if you visit friends and relatives. You don't need special foods or special equipment. You don't have to carry miniature scales with which to weigh out your food. You don't have to eat food which you are not accustomed to eating. You don't have to look for certain types of food. You don't have to carry cumbersome books which give a detailed accounting of the caloric content of different foods. (It's okay to do that if you have interest in what you are eating. It's just not *required* that you do it in order to lose weight.) You can say, "I'm slim and trim," or "I'm full," or "Do I have to eat it all?" wherever you are. You can use the visualizations wherever you are. You can *always* follow the steps in this program.

Not having to change the type of food that you eat as you adjust your weight to a new, lower level is important. Most people aren't going to permanently change the types of foods that they eat. If they grew up in the Northeast, they will eat one type of food. If they grew up in the South or in the West they will eat another type of food. If they have been raised on Italian food, Oriental food, Mexican food or any other type of food, they aren't likely to give it up permanently. That is a redeeming feature of this program of body weight adjustment: it is not necessary to change the type of food that you eat in order to lose weight.

These are some of the features of this method which you will wish to emphasize to someone you are helping.

Things to do during Week Twenty-Nine: Continue to follow the steps of the program just as you have been doing. Record your points daily. When appropriate, record your comments also.

WEEK THIRTY

Comments: Perhaps you have arrived at WEEK THIRTY and find that you need to lose some more weight. That will be easy enough since you have already lost weight. You know that it is just a matter of time before your appestat will have your weight at the level that *you desire*. Since following the steps in the program is easy, continuing is easy. Take consolation in the fact that you are at WEEK THIRTY. Others are just beginning.

By now you have lost 15 to 30 pounds. That should be incentive enough for anyone to continue a weight reduction program. Now you only need to be on guard against distractions.

Should you experience any hint of distractions or complacency, replace them with *repetition*. Repetition is the key to the Appestat Program. If you feel the need to more actively stimulate your appestat to change, repeat the phrases you have been using more often. Repeat them as often as you wish. Say the words, "I am slim and trim. I'm full. Do I *have* to eat it all?" Say them whenever you want to say them. Keep that *image* of a trim you in your mind at all times! Enough repetition will have the information as firmly ingrained in your brain as are the days of the week or the ABCs.

Contemplating the reality of a *permanent* change in one's body weight is exciting. The vision of this forthcoming reality should be coupled with an intense attention to the "now," to the business at hand, to the following of the steps in the program *today*. Why?

Body weight reduction occurs in a stair-step fashion. Initially there is a decrease in weight. The decrease in weight may be followed by a brief plateau. After that the weight decreases again. If you plot your weight loss on a piece of graph paper, the curve will probably look like stair-steps rather than a smooth downward-sloping line. For that reason, if you concentrate on the "now," you won't be distracted by what might have happened yesterday. It won't matter whether you are on a "downward slope" or on a temporary "plateau," because *you will be concentrating on resetting your appestat.*

Whether or not you have reached the weight you desire, it is important for you to stay with this program for another 22 weeks. Think about the steps. Think about the mechanisms involved in resetting the appestat. Why?

If you do concentrate on this program—the steps, the information, the repetitious phrases—for another 22 weeks, that will carry you through all the seasons of the year. Thereafter you will be set. It is important to go through one full cycle of 12 months. There are certain occasions during the year—office parties, club parties, birthdays, Thanksgiving, Christmas, New Year's, picnics, homecomings—when you are "expected" to consume large quantities of food to demonstrate your enjoyment of the occasion. (You can demonstrate your enjoyment of the occasion by commenting on the quality of the food, by noting the skill which might have been required to prepare it, or by making other appropriate observations.) Read *something* from this book before attending a function where you are expected to eat a lot of food.

By going through one full year—and abiding by your *new* appestat setting—you will enjoy the occasions *and* maintain your course toward a new, permanent lower body weight. If you do eat less, you won't notice. If you do eat less and someone else notices, he may or may not comment. That is immaterial. If he does comment, that doesn't mean you have done something that is improper. His comment is just his editorial opinion and nothing more. It should be dismissed as such.

You are free to have the body weight that you wish to have for as long as you wish to have it.

Things to do during Week Thirty: Continue to follow the steps in the program. Follow all of them. Tell yourself that you are "slim and trim," that you're "full," that you "don't have to eat at all." If you have included activity as a part of your program, mention it in your "comments" each day.

ALL OF THE OTHER WEEKS

Comments: If you have carefully followed this program for 30 complete weeks, you have reprogrammed your food intake drives. You have participated in a type of voluntary "brainwashing." You have let your centers for controlling food intake know that your body weight is to be adjusted to a new level. Don't worry if your weight is not there yet. It *will* be! Your weight control center *won't be satisfied* until your weight is controlled at the new level. It's time to celebrate!

Continue to do the mental exercises you have established. Follow them faithfully. Periodically go back and reread the comments associated with the various weeks of the program that you have already completed. This type of mental exercise is good for the nerve circuits you are retraining. Continue to follow the basic steps of the program for *at least* another *22 weeks*. That will take you through one complete year on the program. Thereafter it will be forever fixed in your mind. Beyond one year, continue to follow the steps of the program for as long as you wish—for the rest of your life if you wish.

Here is a real challenge. See if you are up to it. The challenge is not so much in the *doing* as in the *remembering*.

At least once each week during the next 22 weeks visualize yourself, at your new weight, doing things that you enjoy or things that you think you might enjoy if you had the opportunity to do them. (It is going to be a challenge to do it 22 weeks in a row, but once you get into the swing of things, you will find that it is easy to visualize something new each week.) When you do the visualization, include as much detail as possible. Remember to visualize yourself *at your new weight* because that's where you're going to be from now on. Don't *substitute* the visualizations for the steps you have been following. Make them an *addition* to your program. To help you get started, an example is given below:

Picture this in your mind: Your weight is exactly where you want it. You are slim and trim. You wear fashionable clothes. It's fun to dress up and go places.

You are on a vacation. You are on a cruise aboard a ship. You are healthy and energetic. You have the energy to enjoy all of the things associated with your vacation. You go and see things during the day when the ship is in port. You enjoy entertainment in the evenings. You step lively when you move about. Picture yourself taking a brisk stroll along the deck of the ship in the early evening. Your respiratory system, your heart and the other systems of your body feel better than they have ever felt. The aerobic activity of walking in the evening ocean breezes feels good to you! Picture yourself joining friends for dinner later in the evening aboard ship. There are delicious hors d'oeuvres spread about. There are lavish dishes of seafoods and other enticing entrees. There are exotic fruits. What do you do? You enjoy yourself! Your body weight control mechanisms work just as well here as they do at home! You don't have to say to yourself, "I'll go off my diet until I get back home"—then feel guilty because you do. Even worse, you don't have to watch while others enjoy the gourmet fare while you, with iron discipline, think of the tuna and lettuce that you'll eat later. By now you almost subconsciously follow the steps that you have learned. *You* aren't concerned about body weight control. You have given your appestat new instructions. You are going to enjoy yourself while *it* does the job it is *supposed* to do!

The above is just one example of a visualization. You can easily think of others. Visualize yourself, at your new weight, doing things that you enjoy. Get a good mental image of how good it is to do things as the "new" you instead of the "old" you, because *that's the way it's going to be from now on!*

You have a new life ahead of you! Bless you. You deserve it!

References

Brands, B., J. A. Thornhill, M. Hirst and C. W. Gowdey. "Suppression of food intake and body weight gain by naloxone in rats." *Life Sciences* 24:1773–1778, 1979.

Bray, G. A. *The Obese Patient.* Philadelphia: Saunders, 1976.

Douglas, B. H. "Use of visualizations and repetitious phrases to reduce body weight." *Journal of the Mississippi Academy of Sciences* 32:46, 1987.

Douglas B. H., Guyton, A. C., Langston, J. B. and Bishop, V. S. "Hypertension caused by salt loading: II. Fluid volume and tissue pressure changes." *American Journal of Physiology* 207:669–671, 1964.

Douglas, B. H., Clower, B. R. and Williams, W. L. "The effect of pregnancy on dietary-induced cardiovascular damage in RF strain mice." *American Journal of Obstetrics and Gynecology* 102:248–251, 1968.

Dyer, Wayne W. *Your Erroneous Zones.* New York: Avon, 1977.

Farrell, P. A. "Exercise and endorphins—male responses." *Medicine and Science in Sports and Exercise* 17:89–93, 1985.

Food and Nutrition Board. *Recommended Dietary Allowances* (9th rev. ed.), Washington, D.C.: National Academy of Sciences, National Research Council, 1980.

Garrow, J. S. *Energy Balance and Obesity in Man.* Amsterdam: Elsevier/North Holland, 1978.

Grossman, A. "Endorphins and exercise." *Clinical Cardiology* 7:255–260, 1984.

Grossman, A. "Endorphins: Opiates for the masses." *Medicine and Science in Sports and Exercise* 17:101–105, 1985.

Grossman, A. and Sutton, J. R. "Endorphins: What are they? How are they measured? What is their role in exercise?" *Medicine and Science in Sports and Exercise* 17:74–81, 1985.

Harber, V. J., and Sutton, R. R. "Endrophins and exercise." *Sports Medicine* 1:154–171, 1984.

Hirschman, G. H., and Burton, B. T. (Eds.). "Symposium on surgical treatment of morbid obesity." *American Journal of Clinical Nutrition* (Supplement) 33(2):356, 1980.

Kromhout, D., Bosschieter, E. B., and Coulander, C. "The inverse relation between fish consumption and 20-year mortality from coronary Heart Disease." *The New England Journal of Medicine* 312 (19):1205–1209, 1985.

Lew, E. A., and Garfinkel, L. "Variations in mortality by weight among 750,000 men and women." *Journal of Chronic Diseases* 32:563–576, 1979.

Masoro, E. "State of knowledge on action of food restriction on aging." *Basic Life Science* 35:105–116, 1985.

Masoro, E. J. "Aging and nutrition—can diet affect life span?" *Transactions of the Association of Life Insurance Medical Directors of America* 67:30–44, 1985.

McCay, C. M., Crowell, M. F. and Maynard, L. M. "The effect of retarded growth upon the length of life span and upon ultimate body size." *Journal of Nutrition* 10:63–70, 1935.

Morley, John E. "The neuroendocrine control of appetite: The role of the endogenous opiates, cholecystokinin, TRH, Gamma-amino-butyric-acid and the diazepam receptor." *Life Sciences* 27:355–368, 1980.

Morley, John E. and A. S. Levine. "Stress-induced eating is mediated through endogenous opiates." *Science* 209: 1259–1260, 1980.

Paffenbarger, R. S., Jr., Hyde, R. T., Wing, A. L. and Hsieh, C. "Physical activity, all-cause mortality, and longevity of college alumni." *The New England Journal of Medicine* 314(10):605–613, 1986.

Phillipson, B., Rothrock, D. W., Connor, W. E., Harris, W. S., and Illingworth, D. R. "Reduction of plasma lipids, lipoproteins, and apoproteins by dietary fish oils in patients with hypertriglyceridema." *The New England Journal of Medicine* 312 (19):1210–1216, 1985.

Segal, K. R., Gutin, B., Nyman, A. M., Pi-Sunyer, F. X. "Thermic effect of food at rest, during exercise, and after exercise in lean and obese men of similar body weight." *Journal of Clinical Investigation* 76(3):1107–1112, 1985.

Steinberg, H. and Sykes, E. A. "Introduction to Symposium on endorphins and behavioural processes; review of literature on endorphins and exercise." *Pharmacology Biochemistry and Behavior* 23:857–862, 1985.

Tortora, G. J. *Principles of Human Anatomy,* Harper & Row, Publishers, New York, 1986.

van Loon, Hendrik. *The Story of Mankind,* Garden City Publishing, N.Y., 1926.

Whittington-Coleman, P. J., Carrier, O., Jr. and Douglas, B. H. "The effects of propranolol on cholesterol-induced atheromatous lesions." *Atherosclerosis* 18:337–345, 1973.

Wilkins, R. W. and Levinsky, N. G. (Eds.), *Medicine,* 3rd Edition, Little, Brown and Co., Boston, 1983

Willis, J. "How to take weight off (and keep it off) without getting ripped off." *FDA Consumer,* Rockville, Md., Department of Health and Human Services, Publication No. (FDA) 85-1116, 1985.

Yu, B. P., Masoro, E. J., Murata, I. Bertrand, H. A. and Lynd, F. T. "Life span study of SPF Fisher 344 male rats fed ad libitum or restricted diets: Longevity, growth, lean body mass and disease." *Journal of Gerontology* 37:130–141, 1982.

Subject Index

SURVEY

If you will allow us to use your data in our research reports, please send us the following information when you have completed the program: Sex and age, weight at the beginning of the program, weight at the end of the program, and the number of weeks that you were on the program. (Example: Female; 41 years old; 167 pounds, beginning; 117 pounds, ending; 53 weeks on program.)

Include any comments you wish to make and send to:

SURVEY/QRP BOOKS
P.O. BOX 123
BRANDON, MS 39042